Health Care UK 1999/2000

The King's Fund review of health policy

Health Care UK 1999/2000

The King's Fund review of health policy

Edited by John Appleby and Anthony Harrison

King's Fund

Published by
King's Fund Publishing
11–13 Cavendish Square
London W1M 0AN

First published 1999

ISBN 1 85717 287 6

A CIP catalogue record for this book is available from the British Library

Available from:

King's Fund Bookshop
11–13 Cavendish Square
London
W1M 0AN

Tel: 020 7307 2591
Fax: 020 7307 2801

Printed and bound in Great Britain

Cover photo from www.johnbirdsall.co.uk

CONTENTS

POLICY NOTES

POLICY ANALYSIS

DATASCAN

CONTRIBUTORS

John Appleby
Director, Health Systems Programme, King's Fund Policy & Development Directorate

Juan I Baeza
Research Officer, Effective Practice Programme, King's Fund Policy & Development Directorate

Angela Coulter
Director, King's Fund Policy & Development Directorate

Steve Dewar
Fellow, Effective Practice Programme, King's Fund Policy & Development Directorate

Steve Gillam
Director, Primary Care Programme, King's Fund Policy & Development Directorate

Anthony Harrison
Fellow, Health Systems Programme, King's Fund Policy & Development Directorate

John Hayward
Honorary Fellow, Health Systems Programme, King's Fund Policy & Development Directorate

Clare Jenkins
Project Officer, Primary Care Programme, King's Fund Policy & Development Directorate

Justin Keen
Fellow, Health Systems Programme, King's Fund Policy & Development Directorate

Rudolf Klein
Senior Associate, King's Fund

Richard Lewis
Visiting Fellow, Primary Care Programme, King's Fund Policy & Development Directorate

John McClenahan
Fellow in Leadership Development, King's Fund Leadership Development Directorate

Gill Malbon
Research Officer, Primary Care Programme, King's Fund Policy & Development Directorate

Bill New
Independent Health Policy Analyst

Rebecca Rosen
Fellow, Primary Care Programme, King's Fund Policy & Development Directorate

EDITORIALS

Has the NHS a future?

Rudolf Klein

There is a curious paradox at the heart of the Labour Government's policies for the National Health Service. These are designed to strengthen, improve and modernise the NHS, but in the outcome they will add to the pressures for change in the way in which health care is funded and organised in this country. The one monument to old Labour to have survived the purge of inherited dogma and policies – carried out in the name of the Third Way – may over the next decade or so become a candidate for rebuilding as its foundations begin to look increasingly fragile.

This is a large claim to make in the warm afterglow of the NHS's self-congratulatory 50th birthday celebrations and at a time when the Government is increasing the NHS's funding, albeit only modestly. But it rests on two simple propositions. The first is that the Labour Government's policies will generate extra demands on the NHS by raising public expectations. The second is that the Government's centralising policies will increase the political costs of any failure to meet those demands. Rubbing those two propositions together yields a third: unless a future Labour government increases NHS funding to meet rising expectations on a scale hitherto not contemplated – and thereby offends against its proclaimed aim of keeping down both public expenditure and taxes – the Health Service will become an ever heavier political liability. From which it follows that there will be strong incentives to search out a formula for a system of health care which allows governments to wriggle out of this dilemma: of having to choose between ever heavier economic costs or ever greater political costs (and quite possibly having to carry both).

Rising expectations

The notion of rising public expectations – translated into increasing demands on the NHS – is a slippery one. Intuitively, it makes great sense: in a society with rising standards of living (at least for the majority), it seems sensible to assume that the transformation of patients into consumers – a subversive linguistic revolution that has crept up on us over the last decade or so – is transforming attitudes towards health care: that health care consumers will expect to have an ever increasing choice from an ever expanding list of goods delivered to ever improving quality specifications. Moreover, the idea of having to wait for days to see a GP or for weeks for an appointment with a consultant may soon, in a consumer society, seem as outrageously odd as having to go on a waiting list for permission to shop in a supermarket. Add to this the fact of a more educated public with rapidly growing access to information, and the thesis that public expectations are increasing more quickly than the NHS's resources looks remarkably plausible, so creating an ever-widening gap between what is wanted and what is on offer.[1]

This said, the evidence in support of the thesis is remarkably thin. No one has yet measured 'expectations' directly. So we are left searching for indirect evidence, and there clearly is some. More people are spending more money on private health care;[2] over time, dissatisfaction with the NHS appears to have increased. Demand has crept up:[3] a 15 per cent increase in the number of consultations with GPs and a 20 per cent rise in the number of first-time A&E attenders over 10 years[4] – a trend in the expected direction but, with an ageing population, hardly suggesting a dramatic surge in expectations. But there is also evidence on the other side of the argument. In comparative studies, British consumers turn out to be – most surprisingly – as happy with their access to health care and waiting times as those in countries with different and more generously funded systems.[5] The NHS continues to be Britain's most popular institution. Not surprisingly, then, agnosticism seems to be the most appropriate reaction to the assertion that the NHS is suffering from a permanent crisis of 'underfunding'[6] – a somewhat elusive notion, in any case, absent of any precise definition of what the NHS ought to be funded for in the first place.

Shaping demand

So we appear to be left speculating rather inconclusively about the future. But the picture changes if we introduce one further – crucial but frequently ignored – consideration. This is that the NHS is itself shaping expectations and demands. Historically the NHS has been the most successful health care system ever invented for dampening down both expectations and demands, which is why it is also the most effectively parsimonious system. Designed to meet needs as defined by professionals, not to respond to demands from consumers, it was in its conception a model of technocratic paternalism.[7] It was able to draw on a deep reservoir of deference to doctors. Perhaps most important, providers had little or no incentive to raise expectations or encourage demands, which would only create extra work for themselves and bring little or no financial rewards (in sharp contrast to systems operating on a fee for service basis).

Changing dynamics

All this is now changing. Partly the reasons lie in wider social transformations already touched on. The NHS's ability to control expectations has weakened: only consider the explosion of media interest in health care. But the dynamics of the NHS are also changing. The 1991 Conservative model was designed to ensure that money would follow patients – i.e. that there would be incentives to increase activity. If it had worked, there might also have been incentives to pump-up demands. But it did not. However, ironically enough, it is Labour policies that are likely to generate higher expectations and demands, albeit by a different route.

Labour's White Paper[8] is traditional in its use of language. It consistently refers to patients, not consumers. It talks about meeting needs, not demands. It carefully tiptoes around the issue of choice. But the whole thrust of its proposals is that there will be increasing visibility for the performance of local providers. Not only will it be possible to assess their performance against national service frameworks and guidelines produced by the new National Institute for Clinical Excellence, there will also be a stream of comparative information. In short, the gap between the worst and the best performers will be exposed to public scrutiny. In many respects this is a very welcome development (always assuming that it is possible to produce statistics that inform rather than merely alarm or puzzle). In turn, however, the exercise is likely to encourage the expectation that it will be possible, in Nye Bevan's words, 'to generalise the best' – by definition, an impossible policy aim.

Greater visibility

Greater visibility for the performance of the NHS may have a further consequence. This is to give extra impetus to the demystification of the medical profession, a process already accelerated by the Bristol case and other examples of medical blunders. To the extent that doctors will be more accountable for their performance under the new system of clinical governance – supervised by the Government's new inspectorate, the Commission for Health Improvement – so again there will be more visibility for their activities and mistakes. Again, this is a wholly welcome development. But, also, it is likely to weaken the NHS's ability to control expectations, an ability that has depended largely on respect for, and deference to, the medical profession.

Long-term pressures

The catalogue of Labour policies which may bring immediate dividends – and indeed may, individually, be desirable – but which will also add to the long-term pressures on the NHS is longer still. Consider the possible effect on consumer expectations of introducing NHS Direct and walk-in surgeries: might this not (dread thought) actually encourage people to assume that health care should be available on demand? Consider also the financial implications of setting up primary care groups. At first sight setting capped budgets for all PCG activities may seem like a triumph for the Treasury, by bringing prescribing costs under control and making GPs responsible for checking each other's spending patterns. But the long-term effects may be to add to the pressure to increase the NHS's total budget: if PCGs overspend (as they will), they are much more likely to be able to mobilise public support than the managers of health authorities or trusts. The public tends to believe doctors, not managers or politicians, and if GPs proclaim that they have overspent only because of the needs of their patients (not because they are incompetent or extravagant), they are likely to be believed.

So much for the reasons why we should expect the pressures for extra spending to increase at a faster rate than in the past, even without taking into account other much discussed factors: the ageing of the population and the ever expanding menu of what it is technologically possible to do in health care (and the incentives to the pharmaceutical industry to raise public expectations by launching new products). For a Government committed to budgetary austerity, this is an unwelcome prospect. But Labour's own policies have made it more difficult to resist those pressures. They have ensured that the political costs of disappointing expectations or frustrating demands are likely to be even higher than they have been in the past for other governments – like the previous Conservative administration, which was rightly or wrongly perceived to be short-changing health care. Ironically the NHS could yet turn into as much of an incubus for Labour as it proved for the Conservatives.

Ministers appear to be operating under the delusion that they can actually control what happens in the NHS: that, for example, the tide of waiting lists will turn if only they give the command.

Centralisation

Not only are Labour policies generating higher expectations – they also firmly put ministers centre stage, directly responsible for satisfying those expectations. This flows from the centralising thrust of Labour's programme of reform. In many respects, Labour's new NHS represents a reversion to a command and control model. Not only are there to be national standards, but the Secretary of State for Health will control the implementation of those standards, through the new Institute and Commission. Where previous governments have sought to pursue a blame diffusion strategy – by stressing the importance of local decisions about what services to provide in the light of judgements about local needs – Labour is pursuing a policy of blame-concentration. Ministers appear to be operating under the delusion that they can actually control what happens in the NHS: that, for example, the tide of waiting lists will turn if only they give the command. Consequently, if things go wrong, if standards are not achieved, if services fall short of expectations, there will be no ambiguity about who carries the blame: the Secretary of State. And the effect will be compounded if it turns out that the Secretary of State's decision to limit the use of Viagra proves to be a precedent for the future, and if central government takes responsibility, for the first time ever, for explicit rationing decisions and so gives dramatic visibility to resource constraints which in the past were blurred by being left to individual clinical decisions. In short, the prospect is one of ever-increasing political overload, as economic parsimony becomes ever more expensive politically.

The future

It is just conceivable that the Chancellor of the Exchequer will show unprecedented generosity in funding the NHS to meet expanding expectations. Just conceivably, too, the dynamics of the new NHS may generate an increase in activity to match rising demands. But a more realistic scenario may be to see a second-term Labour Government having second thoughts about its commitment to the NHS in its present form, as distinct from a commitment to the principle of ensuring access to health care for the whole population. A minimalist strategy might be to shift responsibility for health care to the English regions, on the Scandinavian model: the snag being that it is difficult to see how this would achieve genuine devolution if the regions remained financially dependent on central government. A maximalist strategy might be to move towards a social insurance system on the Dutch or German model, incorporating both for-profit insurers and a national social insurance scheme, with the government concentrating on a regulatory rather than funding or provider role.

Alternatives

There is, then, no shortage of alternative models – all of which seem to perform at least as well as the NHS in most respects. But before engaging in a model building exercise (which, in any case, is premature) it may be better to engage in a debate about the principles that ought to inform the choice of models. First, almost any alternative model is likely to be more expensive than the NHS, even though it may make fewer demands on the taxpayer: should this be considered as a drawback (higher administrative and other costs) or an advantage (bringing in extra resources)? Secondly, how much importance should be attached to choice of GPs and specialists – the effective lack of such choice for most people for most of the time being one of the distinguishing characteristics of the NHS? If high priority is to be attached to this as a long-term policy aim – in line with the aspirations of a consumerist society – what price are we prepared to pay in terms of creating the spare capacity needed to bring it about? Thirdly, although much is made of inequalities within the NHS, the largest source of inequality in health care stems from the differential ability of people to buy into the private sector. But health policy continues to be made as though the private sector did not exist. If the role of the private sector was recognised, it might be possible to address the more interesting question of what inequalities should count as inequities in health care[9] and how to make the best of what is inescapably a two-tier health care system. Finally, the NHS stands on three legs: universality, freedom from payment at the point of delivery and comprehensiveness of coverage. Can all three policy objectives be pursued or will the price of maintaining the first two be continued shrinkage of coverage – the pattern so far? And is that the most appropriate trade-off?

Given Labour's present stance, all this may seem redundantly speculative. But that stance could alter rapidly once the economic and political costs of present policies become apparent. New Labour is not a society for the preservation of old Labour monuments. And while Conservative iconoclasm in health care policy was always constrained by the public perception that the Tories could not be trusted on this issue, a Labour Government may be able to be more radical precisely because it carries no legacy of distrust.

REFERENCES

1. Thwaite B. *Foundation Lecture*. University of Southampton: Institute of Health Policy Studies, 1987.

2. Laing W. *Laing's Review of Private Healthcare 1998*. London: Laing and Buisson Publications, 1998.

3. Mulligan JA and Judge K. Public Opinion and the NHS. In: Harrison A, editor. *Health Care UK*. London: King's Fund, 1997.

4. Secretary of State for Health. *Department of Health: Departmental Report*. London: HMSO, 1999.

5. Donelan K, Blendon RJ, Schoen C *et al*. The cost of health system change: public discontent in five nations. *Health Affairs* 1999; 18 (3): 206–16.

6. Dixon J and Harrison A. Funding the NHS: A little local difficulty? *BMJ* 1997; 314: 216–19.

7. Klein R. *The New politics of the NHS*. London: Longman, 1995.

8. Secretary of State for Health. *The New NHS: Modern-Dependable*. London: HMSO, 1997.

9. Klein R. Acceptable Inequalities. In: Green D, editor. *Acceptable Inequalities?* London: Institute of Economic Affairs, 1988.

Can NICE influence the diffusion of new technologies?

Rebecca Rosen

The desire to influence the introduction of new medical technologies – restricting the diffusion of unproven or ineffective interventions and promoting the use of those which are effective – is evident in the proposed appraisal role for the National Institute of Clinical Excellence (NICE). But how will NICE face the challenge – illustrated recently by Viagra – of interpreting evidence of effectiveness in the light of political pressures created by scarce resources, public demand and clinician and media advocacy? What will happen to the many new technologies that are not the subject of NICE appraisals? And how will clinicians and commissioners respond to NICE recommendations at a local level?

Appraisal

NICE plans to appraise 30 to 50 technologies each year, some of which will be identified through the new NHS Centre for Horizon Scanning, and still be under development.[1] With development well underway of new drugs targeted at specific tissues; gene, cell and tissue therapies; and new surgical and radiological techniques, there will be no shortage of new interventions as candidates for appraisal. Technologies will be chosen for appraisal on the basis of predicted clinical or cost impact, and the manufacturers of selected technologies will be informed prior to their launch of the need to provide evidence of effectiveness to the NICE appraisal committee. If the emerging technology is a surgical technique, research may have to be commissioned by the Department of Health.[2]

Exact data requirements are still under discussion but will include a descriptive account of the intervention, the epidemiology of relevant indications and target patient groups, cost-effectiveness data, details of aggregate cost impact to the NHS, and any data relating to equity. Details of research methods and outcome measures used will also be required.

National guidance

The appraisals will be conducted by a multidisciplinary group in consultation with relevant experts and patient groups. Methods for judging the data and developing policy recommendations have not yet been described, but the group will use the data to recommend use or restriction of the technology before widespread diffusion occurs. This explicit and systematic process will produce timely and authoritative *national* guidance. However, certain characteristics of new medical technologies make it particularly difficult to develop effective, evidence-based policy.

First, new surgical and equipment technologies are often dynamic – continuing to evolve and develop for some time after they are launched. Gelijns and Rosenberg[3] illustrate this point with reference to early endoscopes, which caused some severe complications until a 'cold tip' light source was developed which did not burn through tissue. This modification dramatically altered the balance of risks and benefits associated with the technique, rendering previous research findings obsolete. Although many new technologies undergo more subtle modifications after their launch, the changes are often made in response to problems experienced by early users and will tend to improve outcomes. Conversely, as technologies diffuse into routine use on less carefully selected patients, the outcomes obtained may not reach the standards reported in teaching hospital-based efficacy studies.

Rapid change

Thus the results of early technology assessments may soon lose their authority as a basis for guidance on initial use. NICE will undertake periodic reappraisals, but with the rapid transfer of information between countries, overseas use of new technologies could result in improved outcomes and strong public demand for interventions that are banned or restricted to research in the UK. The appraisal system could get bogged-down if the need for an early reappraisal delays work on other emerging technologies.

Secondly, the consultation document on NICE appraisals does not discuss potential problems with the integrity of data provided by manufacturers about their own products. The acceptability to local clinicians of recommendations to the NHS on appropriate use may be undermined if there is controversy about the quality of the research on which the recommendations are based. While there is an expectation that NICE guidance *will* be implemented locally, it is not yet clear what will happen if local clinicians do not comply with the guidance.

While there is an expectation that NICE guidance will be implemented locally, it is not yet clear what will happen if local clinicians do not comply with the guidance.

Technology creep

Thirdly, and perhaps the greatest challenge for the NHS, is 'technology creep' or the application of existing technologies to new groups of patients or new diseases. This remains one of the most inexplicit processes in health care, led by individual clinicians in response to the needs of individual patients and rarely linked, at the early stages, to evaluative research. The capacity to identify – let alone control – technology creep is limited and the process often comes to light only when departmental budgets are overspent as a result. If creeping applications of new technologies are not subject to NICE appraisals, there are few incentives within clinical settings – where an individual patient perspective predominates – to evaluate whether new uses of a technology offer value for money to the local population.

This population perspective was more typically taken by health authorities, some of which have tried – with limited success – to link the use of selected new technologies to evidence of effectiveness. But health authority staff have barely been able to keep abreast of technology creep and innovation in their local providers and few have had the resources to manage the detailed negotiations and contracting required to shape technology adoption.[4] Furthermore, their capacity for detailed work on new technologies is limited by a falling staff complement, and much of their attention is currently focused on supporting the development of PCGs.

PCGs will be faced with new technologies – with or without NICE guidance – in both their provider and their commissioner roles. However, given their overwhelming workload, they will not necessarily prioritise work to influence technology diffusion. Furthermore, with the demise of the internal market and the fragmentation of commissioning decisions between numerous small PCGs, it is now much harder to exert political or financial leverage over trusts in relation to their use of new technologies.

Systematic approach

Despite these potential implementation difficulties, NICE will offer a systematic and transparent approach to evaluating new technologies before they diffuse widely. Mowatt *et al.*[5] argued that the evaluation of new technologies should be started early and be iterative in nature. The link between the Centre for Horizon Scanning and the NICE appraisal process certainly offers a system to do this and to produce timely guidance which will end the so-called 'postcode rationing' that has dogged the launch of many new technologies. However, the evolving nature of most technologies and their applications means that producing the guidance with periodic reappraisals will not be the endpoint. NICE may also have to take an active role in managing post-launch research programmes to ensure that an appropriate balance is achieved between efficacy studies and effectiveness research, and to monitor and act upon changes in the cost-effectiveness of new technologies as they become established.

A new attitude

Finally, for all those new technologies not covered by NICE appraisals, the successful development and implementation of clinical governance probably offers the best chance for promoting the research-linked, evidence-based introduction of effective new technologies. If clinical governance succeeds in fostering a new culture and attitude to clinical quality, then on-going questioning and evaluation of the effectiveness of new technologies would become more the norm than at present. This may have its greatest impact in relation to hospital clinicians who drive forward the introduction of most non-drug new technologies. Hospital decisions on new technologies are often dominated by consideration of their likely impact on reputation, staff recruitment and clinician satisfaction rather than on clinical outcome. Incorporating a rigorous review of evidence of effectiveness into decisions about adopting new technologies represents a modest but attainable aspiration for life after NICE and clinical governance.

REFERENCES

1. Rawlins M. In pursuit of quality: the National Institute for Clinical Excellence. *Lancet* 1999; 353: 1079–82.

2. NHS Executive. *Faster Access to 'Modern Treatment': How will NICE appraisal work. A discussion paper*. Leeds: NHSE, 1999.

3. Gelijns AC, Rosenberg N. The dynamics of technological change in medicine. *Health Affairs* 1994; 13: 28–46.

4. Rosen R, Mays N. The impact of the UK NHS purchaser–provider split on the 'rational' introduction of new medical technologies. *Health Policy* 1998; 43: 103–23.

5. Mowatt G *et al. When and How to Assess Fast-Changing Technologies: a comparative study of medical applications of four generic technologies*. Southampton: University of Southampton, 1997.

A future for primary care groups?

Richard Lewis, Gill Malbon and Steve Gillam

The creation of primary care groups (PCGs) and primary care trusts (PCTs) lies at the heart of The New NHS – the Labour Government's plans for reorganising health services. PCGs have been operational only since April 1999 and the first PCTs are not due until April 2000. Despite their infant status, PCGs face a challenging agenda and have been put firmly in the 'driving seat' by the Government. New organisational forms have been introduced and the internal market discarded. There is much about The New NHS that looks familiar, which is hardly surprising given the Government's concerns to avoid knee-jerk reform and to preserve 'what works'. However, there is also much that signals a new departure in the planning and management of health policy. PCGs display characteristics of both continuity and change.1 Local professionals are tasked with planning the use of specialist services, budget-holding by GPs has been extended and the financial incentives for GPs to make 'savings' remain within the new PCGs. There are also other ways in which PCGs build on, rather than replace, the existing policy framework.

Diversification

The evolution of PCGs will hasten the diversification of new roles in primary care. The role of the 'clinician manager' within primary care has been developed through the resource management responsibilities of GP fundholding and later GP commissioning pilots. Within PCGs a new cadre of GPs and community nurses – corporate clinicians – will combine senior management duties with hands-on patient care. Successful PCG chief executives will raise the status of primary care for Health Service managers generally. New kinds of clinical director, combining educational experience and understanding of the performance management agenda, will be needed to advance clinical governance. The latter role and the continuing need for new models of primary care in inner cities present further opportunities for extending the role of primary care nurses.

PCGs will also become the main channel for quality assurance through their responsibilities for managing clinical governance programmes. While clinical governance is new, it is firmly within the tradition of professional self-regulation that has underpinned the management of clinical services for so long. However, it is still not clear how quality standards are to be enforced within the PCG beyond peer exhortation, another similarity with the pre-Labour NHS.

Competition

Elements of competition enshrined within the internal market remain. The purchaser–provider split is a feature of *The New NHS*. The opportunity for PCGs and PCTs to drive down costs by moving (or threatening to move) service agreements between alternative providers has been protected.

The New NHS has also maintained continuity by ensuring that the 'non-cash limited' resources for general practice remain subject to the national GP contract and not the local PCG. Thus, the much vaunted 'unified budget' that is held by each PCG in practice fails to unify total health resources for a given locality. Ironically, it is only through the use of personal medical services (PMS) pilots, an innovation of the previous government, that a unified budget can be created.[2]

Financial incentives

PCGs/PCTs are continuing the focus on financial incentives by agreeing that any savings made under the new scheme will be shared 50-50 by the individual practice and the PCG. General practitioners are being allowed to carry over their fundholding savings, either with agreement with their PCG or by taking a proportion of their savings each year for up to four years. However, there are also a number of ways in which PCGs represent an important departure for the NHS, and primary care in particular. As Health Service organisations, PCGs are 'inclusive' (i.e. the membership of GPs is compulsory). This is in contrast to other recent primary care developments such as GP fundholding, total purchasing pilots and PMS pilots.

The creation of PCGs also redefines the relationship of GPs to each other. Notwithstanding the existing culture that values independence and small organisations, PCGs require collective responsibility. PCGs will have a strategic plan and a single budget that must be managed. GPs that fail to comply with PCG policies may compromise the services available for the patients of their colleagues. However, PCGs have little 'leverage' over recalcitrant GPs at local level. This may be compensated for by a number of important 'top-down' initiatives: the introduction of NICE, CHI, the performance assessment framework and the national service frameworks may assist PCGs in developing more consistency in the delivery of clinical services.

GPs that fail to comply with PCG policies may compromise the services available for the patients of their colleagues. However, PCGs have little 'leverage' over recalcitrant GPs at local level.

New relationships

PCGs have also created the potential for new strategic relationships, both within primary care and beyond. Board membership is clearly laid down by the NHS Executive (although with some local discretion given to medical members of the PCG). This suggests that the policy objective of 'integration' is now to be pursued through regulation rather than simple exhortation. The mandatory appointment of nurses to PCG boards and the opportunity to appoint more widely to PCT boards represent formal power sharing between primary care professionals (within the context of a built-in medical majority). Similarly, guaranteed board membership for local authority representatives and lay members suggests a more structured approach to public involvement and multi-agency collaboration than has been achieved through previous initiatives such as fundholding and total purchasing. Whether this attempt at power sharing proves real or illusory is an important issue for the evaluation of PCGs.

WHAT DO PCGs NEED NOW?

Both the total purchasing pilots (TPPs) and the GP commissioning group initiatives were extensively evaluated and provide useful hints for PCG and PCT development. Clearly, there are differences between PCGs and their predecessors, notably the inclusive nature of PCGs/PCTs and the wider group involvement. However, TPPs and GP commissioning do provide relevant learning.

The organisational challenge faced by PCGs/PCTs has been much discussed,[3] and pointers for success have been repeatedly listed:[4, 5]

- a strong executive

management team with the mandate to take strategic decisions on behalf of the wider group
- the development of a clear vision and agenda for action
- an inclusive approach leading to the development of collective responsibility and corporacy
- sophisticated project management capacity
- investment in clinical and management information systems
- ability to engage effectively and create partnerships with external organisations
- adequate resourcing of organisational and management arrangements.

It seems likely that much of PCGs/PCTs' first three years will be spent in organisational development, establishing the teams and the processes to underpin their core functions.

Local interest

New primary care organisations are encouraged to begin developing services in which there is local interest, before moving on to more challenging areas as they gain experience. Conventional wisdom suggests that PCGs/PCTs will make most progress in those roles most familiar to general practitioners. With the concurrent emphasis on clinical governance and the onward march of revalidation, PCGs/PCTs should make progress ironing out some of the glaring variations in the quality of services available at practice level. GP commissioning groups cut their collective teeth on prescribing and, given the financial incentives, this is an area within which PCGs/PCTs should make early progress also. Total purchasing pilots looked to extend their primary health care teams to promote service integration (for example, by employing community psychiatric nurses to reduce unnecessary use of secondary care or tracker nurses to rationalise discharge planning). However, the evidence base to underpin such investments is slim and PCGs/PCTs will need support in collecting, pooling and sharing experience of 'what works'.

The medium term

The New NHS White Paper laid down a model of primary care-based commissioning that was to be universalised. However, in effect, a plurality of different models will operate (within a mixed economy). At present, it is difficult to predict how long it will be before all PCGs are ready for level four. It is possible that some PCGs will never want to take this step. A number of new models may evolve:

- Reluctant PCT: primary care developer, whose prime interest continues to be in developing primary care provision
- Basic PCT: stand-alone purchasing trusts (incremental advance on GP commissioning groups and TPPs, with general practitioners operating under national contract)
- Mid-range PCT: purchaser/ provider offering full range of community services/ intermediate care
- Advanced PCT: purchaser/ provider offering full range of community services/intermediate care, plus PMS. GPs working to local contracts: the UK HMO model.

Support

As Figure 1 shows, primary care organisations within the local health economy will not work in isolation. Advanced PCTs may provide services to neighbouring PCTs; they may also act as a central support system, providing centralised management/ administration/ practice and professional development/education through the community trust on behalf of satellite neighbouring PCGs/ PCTs.

While PCTs undertake these roles, what responsibilities will local health authorities have? Our model suggests that they could end up acting mainly in a strategic role, co-ordinating the provision of highly specialised services. We may see the development of primary care and public health agencies, organised at health authority level or across health authority areas, supporting selected PCGs/PCTs. A further role will be to mitigate a possible 'inverse care' effect as PCGs/PCTs develop at different rates – particularly those with less commissioning experience – containing smaller practices in more deprived areas. This will require health authorities to target resources.

FIGURE 1

PRIMARY CARE WITHIN A LOCAL HEALTH ECONOMY

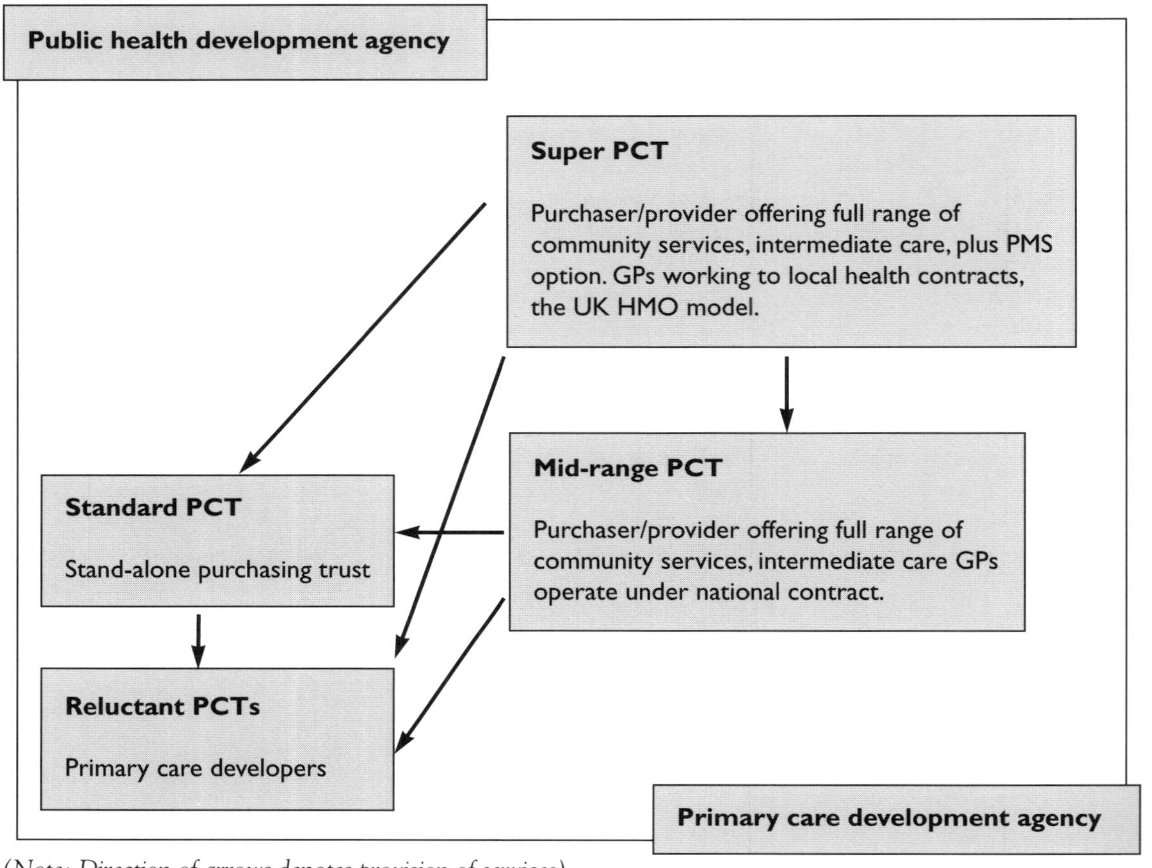

(Note: Direction of arrows denotes provision of services)

THE FUTURE?

A step-wise approach to PCG/PCT development implies a journey, but what is its ultimate destination? The future of the national GP contract is of fundamental importance to the development of PCTs. While GPs remain governed by the 'Red Book' there will inevitably be funding inequities between PCTs and their lines of accountability will be divided.

One obvious destination is that of a UK-style health maintenance organisation (HMO). Much has been written about HMOs and their variants, and together with 'managed care', they present a sometimes confusing array of models. However, they exhibit a number of key characteristics:

- single budget for universal health care for a given population
- management of financial risk within a single entity
- incentive to promote health as well as treat disease
- choice within the organisation to provide service or to commission
- directive control of clinical activity via evidence-based guidelines, audit and utilisation reviews.

PCTs have the potential to emulate health maintenance

TABLE 1

COMPARISON OF HMO AND PCT CHARACTERISTICS

HMO type	*PCT level four (Basic)*	*PCT level four plus PCG-wide PMS (Advanced)*
Unified budget	Unified budget: commissioning hospital and community health services, prescribing and GP support services	Unified budget: commissioning hospital and community health services, prescribing, GP support services and primary care services
Managing financial risk	Managing risk for HCHS and prescribing budgets	Additional risk for primary care (element of personal risk holding by GPs)
Incentive to promote health as well as treat disease	Externally imposed by HA and NHSE to deliver against HImPs	Externally imposed by HA and NHSE to deliver against HImPs
Providers and/or commissioners	Limited opportunity to substitute secondary care for primary care	Unlimited opportunity
Formalised processes of utilisation review and quality assurance	Use of guidelines, audit encouraged through clinical governance and NICE	More stringent peer review, link to contractual stipulations

organisations in a number of important ways, particularly if the general practices associated with the PCT are also personal medical services (PMS) pilots. PCTs will have direct control over increasingly comprehensive budgets and will be able to decide whether to provide care directly or to commission it. PCTs will hold the financial risk relating to performance, and, in the case of the PMS pilots, this risk may extend to the personal incomes of general practitioners. Clinicians within PCTs are likely to be subject to collective agreements about clinical practice augmented by central direction via NICE and national service frameworks. PCTs will be paid to promote healthy lifestyles and prevent disease. These will be bolstered by the requirement to deliver health improvement targets, contained within their HImP.

Finally, PCTs also offer the potential for unifying budgets for health and social care. The integration of community health and social care agencies harks back to arrangements that existed before 1974. *Plus ça change!*

REFERENCES

1. Mays N, Goodwin N. Primary Care Groups in England. In: Klein R, editor. *Implementing the White Paper: Pitfalls and Opportunities*. London: King's Fund, 1998.

2. Lewis R, Gillam S, editors. *Transforming Primary Care*. London: King's Fund, 1999.

3. Mays N, Goodwin N, Killoran A, Malbon G on behalf of the Total Purchasing National Evaluation Team. *Total purchasing: a step towards primary care groups*. London: King's Fund, 1998.

4. Killoran A, Mays N, Wyke S and Malbon G on behalf of the Total Purchasing National Evaluation Team. *Total purchasing. A step towards new primary care organisations*. London: King's Fund, 1999.

5. Wyke S, Mays N, Abbott S, Bevan G, Goodwin N, Killoran A, Malbon G, McLeod H, Posnett J, Raftery J, Robinson R on behalf of the Total Purchasing National Evaluation Team. *Developing Primary Care in The New NHS: Lessons from total purchasing.*

POLICY REVIEW

Anthony Harrison

Part 1 Main Events

Our 1997/98 Health Policy Review described the 'massive range of new policies' announced by the Labour Government in the 15 months since it came to power. In this year's Review, the focus switches from announcement to implementation. Most of this Part will therefore describe how far the new Government's policy proposals have advanced towards having an impact on how the NHS works and, beyond that, on its users.

It has been more than 18 months since the publication of *The New NHS*, and in many areas there has been no change 'on the ground'. Some of the White Paper's proposals required new legislation. It was not until January 1999 that the Health Bill was published, and not until June that it received Royal Assent. Similarly, it was not until July 1999 that the public health White Paper *Saving Lives* was published, following-up, and in some areas expanding on, the proposals made in the 1998 Green Paper *Our Healthier Nation.*

In a small number of areas, new ideas have emerged without being foreshadowed in any white or green paper (for example, the proposal for walk-in primary care centres) and other areas, such as NHS Direct, have developed more rapidly than expected. If, in other respects, the actual pace of change is slow, for those on the ground the timetable to get the new organisations in place and new working relationships established has seemed extremely tight. Last year we reported that the Government had virtually succeeded in getting primary care groups designated by the end of July. This year they are, in principle, up and running, with many looking ahead to becoming primary care trusts. But, as we shall see below, they are faced with a series of new and demanding tasks, which most have little experience of tackling. The same is true for the rest of the NHS, including its central management. So, although Labour's new NHS was intended to build on the old, in practice – like its Conservative predecessor – it is moving the NHS into areas where experience and knowledge are limited.

1.1 Labour's new NHS

The New NHS has subjected the health service to a demanding programme of change. Despite a drive for centralisation, however, different parts of the NHS continue to develop at different speeds and in different ways.

The timetable for implementing the White Paper proposals was set out in July 1998 in *Better Health and Better Health Care: the Next Steps* (HSC 1998/121). According to the Circular, 'the new structures and processes should make it easier to deliver the core agenda', which was described as being:

- *improving health and reducing inequality*
- *providing integrated services*
- *improving quality and responsiveness, and raising standards*
- *improving performance and efficiency*
- *enabling staff to maximise their contribution*
- *improving public confidence in the NHS and social services.* (HSC 1998/121, p.4)

The Circular goes on to suggest that:

> *The approach which must underlie all of this work is:*
> - *to keep each change as simple as possible*
> - *to roll out change, laying sound foundations, building on initial progress in a phased and purposeful way, sharing and learning from emerging good practice, and above all*
> - *to use each change to make a visible difference to patients and communities, on selected issues at first but widening over time.* (HSC 1998/121, p.5)

The generality of the agenda and the banality of the advice might suggest to some that the links between the changes being made and the desired outcomes are not as self-evident as the Circular suggests. It will be some time before such a suspicion can be confirmed by evidence of performance on the ground. In the meantime, as in the early years of the Conservatives' 'new NHS', the process of putting new pieces on the NHS chess board and introducing new rules of the game has absorbed the energies of those charged with making the required changes. In the rest of this Section, therefore, it is administrative change and the accompanying rhetoric that dominate.

PRIMARY CARE GROUPS

By summer 1998, the Government had more or less achieved its target of having the number and the geographical coverage of primary care groups defined. The size of the groups varies considerably, the smallest being responsible for some 46,000 patients and the largest over one-quarter of a million (see Table 1.1).

As the Audit Commission pointed out (*PCGs: an early view of primary care groups in England*, 1999), these variations may be important for how well the groups will perform:

- small PCGs may lack the 'purchasing power' to influence trusts unless they commission services jointly with other PCGs
- conversely, the larger the PCG, the more varied the communities it is likely to contain; thus, large PCG especially, will need to find ways of becoming aware of all local needs and of responding to them
- health authorities will be able to provide more focused support if they are responsible for fewer and larger PCGs, especially if each group has a similar range of devolved responsibilities
- PCGs that contain a large number of smaller

TABLE 1.1

LIST SIZE OF PRIMARY CARE GROUPS IN ENGLAND (1999)

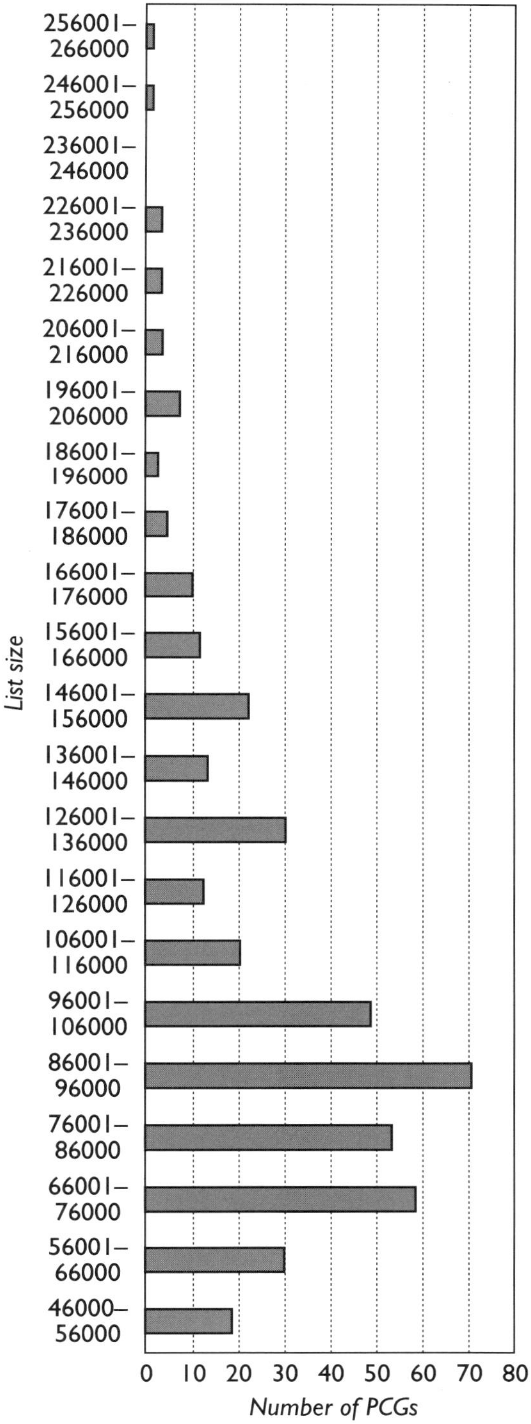

> **BOX 1.1:**
> **PRIMARY CARE IN SCOTLAND, WALES AND NORTHERN IRELAND**
>
> The arrangements described here apply only to England. In Wales, similar arrangements apply but they are called local health groups. In Northern Ireland it seems likely that general practitioners will also act as budgetholders but the precise arrangements had not been determined at the time of writing. In Scotland, however, all forms of general practitioner commissioning have ended. Instead, from 1 April 1999, all care outside hospital will be financed through, and supplied by, primary care trusts. GPs may advise the trusts on commissioning through local health co-operatives, which will have limited budgets for prescribing and the provision of general medical services.

GP practices may find it more difficult to build relationships

- having to work with more than one local authority will also make for complexity for a minority of PCGs. (p.7)

Formally, the groups assumed their new responsibilities as from 1 April 1999, but in practice the speed with which they were created meant that most appear to have focused on getting established rather than setting about the substantive tasks they were faced with. Experience from the 'old regime' suggests that simply getting established is no small task (see Box 1.2).

BOX 1.2: OVERALL LESSONS FOR PCGs

In 1998 a process of evaluating GP commissioning pilots (part of the Policy Research Programme) began. The results of this work carried out at the University of Birmingham suggest that it will take a considerable time for most PCGs to address the tasks they have been set. In particular, the research team found that:

PCGs will tend to focus on issues of structure and process in their early days, as they establish themselves as effective organisations.

Not surprisingly it also found that:

the time commitment for clinical staff is considerable and the impact on practices and NHS trusts will need to be assessed and kept under review;
high quality dedicated management support will be a vital prerequisite to PCG working;
IM&T is more complex and time-consuming than PCGs may at first imagine and will require significant attention by groups.

Moreover, the right organisational structure will take time to identify and develop:

PCGs will need to determine arrangements for carrying out both strategic and operational work, and this may entail structures of a greater complexity than simply the PCG board; there are many personal and organisational development needs to be addressed by PCGs, including work on team building and effective board working.

Furthermore, the groups will be the focus of a series of tensions – between professions, between organisations and between professionals and the public – that will be hard to manage.

nurses are enthusiastic about involvement in PCGs, but groups will need to determine ways of ensuring that they are able to participate in decision-making on an equal basis with GPs;
the health authority/PCG dynamic is of particular importance to the effective development and functioning of the PCG;
user and public involvement presents a real challenge for PCGs and is likely to remain a good intention unless there is clear guidance and support for groups about models of good practice in this area.

Source: adapted from Regen E *et al. First off the Starting Blocks: summary report.* Birmingham: University of Birmingham, 1999, p.6.

According to *The New NHS Modern and Dependable: developing primary care groups* (HSC 1998/139, 13 August 1998), the substantive tasks they have to tackle are:

- *improving the health of, and addressing health inequalities in, their community*
- *developing primary care and community services across the Primary Care Group*
- *advising on, or commissioning directly, a range of hospital services for patients within their area which appropriately meets patients' needs*. (HSC 1998/139, p.6)

Each of these comprises a range of substantial tasks in their own right. According to the Circular, the first includes identification of health needs, contributing to and informing the development of the local health improvement programme (see below), working closely with social services and involving the public in the work of the group so as to inform the delivery of appropriate services.

The second involves service development, reducing variations in the provision of primary care services, improving the quality and standard of the care provided to patients through the development of clinical governance and integrating the delivery of primary and community health services.

The third requires the commissioning of effective and high-quality health services, monitoring the performance of providers of services against the service agreements and contributing to the national drive to reduce waiting lists and times.

Underpinning all of the above is the requirement that each PCG should prepare a three-year investment plan, on an annual cycle, which in turn must be linked to and consistent with the local health improvement programme. The plan, according to *The new NHS Modern and Dependable: primary care groups; delivering the agenda* (HSC 1998/228, 8 December 1998), summarises the intentions for the development of primary care in each area and sets out 'how cost-effective practice based services ... are to be handled during the coming year.'

To carry out these demanding tasks, the groups will have only very modest resources at their disposal. Their management cost allowances have been set at a low level – £3 per head per year – but as they take on more health authority functions that will grow. However, even if they eventually enjoy similar management cost allowances to health authorities – less than £10 per head – they will have much less available than the total purchasing pilots, the organisational form closest to them, some of which enjoyed £6–8 per head in their own right (i.e. over and above health authority costs). The greater size of PCGs means that they should enjoy some scale economies. On the other hand, experience with total purchasing pilots suggests that the task of co-ordinating GPs gives rise to extra management and transaction costs as the numbers involved rise.

Unhappily, the Circular does not offer detailed guidance as to how to discharge each of the tasks it identifies. It seems unlikely that the resources to do the tasks justice will be available. The Birmingham work cited above, as well as the findings of the National Evaluation of Total Purchasing Pilots (Mays N *et al. Total Purchasing: A step towards Primary Care Groups*. London: King's Fund, 1998), suggest that in practice only small parts of the agenda can be tackled at any one time. In part this is because of resource limits, in part because change requires human qualities such as leadership and diplomacy, which are also in short supply, and in part because the knowledge and understanding required are lacking. So, no ready-made solutions are to hand for easy application. The prospect, therefore, is that change will occur at noticeably different rates in different areas and that different issues will be addressed.

TRUSTS

The New NHS foreshadowed only one major change in the organisational framework for the delivery of services – the creation of primary care trusts. As these were one of the Government's proposals that required legislation, there was no substantive move towards bringing them into being during the year. In February 1999, however, the Health Minister, John Denham, issued a paper setting out the nature of the benefits that the new form of trust is expected to bring, as well as an outline of the organisational framework within which they are to operate.

In a letter to all chairs and chief executives of trusts, health authorities and primary care groups in February 1999, the Minister affirmed that primary care trusts will provide:

- *better support to practices which are the cornerstone of the NHS and patient care;*
- *better support to individual clinicians in providing more effective care;*
- *more integrated services, particularly between general practice and community services;*
- *better access, identifying for example where more locally based services should be developed;*
- *decision-making closer to patients, shaped by the professionals who most often meet their needs.*

The paper attached to the letter, *Primary Care Groups*, sets out four 'key principles underlying the new form of Trust':

- *put primary care professionals in the driving seat;*
- *provide public accountability;*
- *support public involvement, with Trusts rooted firmly in the local community;*
- *ensure probity, with robust safeguards both to protect public funds and primary care professionals from suggestions of any conflicts of interest.*

The trusts will have substantial annual budgets – at least £60 million – and considerable discretion over the deployment of these. They will also exercise considerable influence over the development of primary care, including physical investment in new facilities. As the paper notes, no other NHS body will have the same range of flexibilities and opportunities. The reverse side of the coin is that new accountability arrangements will be required (we look at those in Section 2.3).

The New NHS envisaged a staged development from primary care groups to primary care trusts. The Health Act 1999 provides for primary care trusts to take a variety of forms, in particular that there will be a clear distinction between commissioning only and commissioning and providing. The move from one to the other will be subject to consultation and to the Secretary of State, as will their initial establishment. When making his announcement, the Minister made it clear that 'the development of PCTs will be based on local consensus and agreement'. At the time of the Minister's announcement nearly 50 per cent of primary care groups had expressed an interest in becoming primary care trusts.

In contrast, where the statutory framework for change was already in place, as with the primary care pilots – which like trusts are largely focused on the delivery of health care services – change could take place 'on the ground'. By the time last year's Review was written, the first wave of pilots had been approved. The first 'Modernising Primary Care' announcement (PR 1999/0092, 18 February 1999) stated that there were 85 pilots underway covering some 800,000 people. A further wave is under consideration (see the article by Clare Jenkins). As she points out, some of the pilots cut across the structure of primary care groups, and are therefore perhaps best seen as pilots for the sort of services and organisational arrangements that primary care trusts may comprise.

Finally, mergers brought change within the existing trust framework for hospital and community health services. The prime aim of such mergers has been reduction in management costs. However, as John McClenahan points out below, there are reasons for suspecting that the expected gains may not materialise.

HEALTH AUTHORITIES

As noted last year, it is intended that health authorities retain a number of key tasks and (as primary care groups remain in formal terms authority committees) they retain overall responsibility for all purchasing activity. Moreover, as and when primary care groups move on to trust status, authorities will still have overall responsibility for the development of health improvement programmes. These can be seen as the key administrative process that brings together the various elements of the local health economy. The process of 'bringing things together' will be underpinned by a new duty of co-operation introduced in the Health Act 1999, which simply states that 'It is the duty of Health Authorities, Special Health Authorities, Primary Care Trusts and NHS Trusts to co-operate with each other in exercising their functions'.

According to *Health Improvement Programmes: planning for better health and health care* (HSC 1998/167, 5 October 1998), health improvement programmes are 'the local plan of action to improve health and modernise services' which:

> *will replace the fragmentation of the NHS internal market with a coherent planning process within the local health care system and with local authorities and other partner organisations [and] ensure that strategic planning is shaped by the local perspectives and knowledge that PCGs, local government and local communities can bring to bear.* (HSC 1998/167, Guidance, p.1)

Thus the plans are seen as an integrating mechanisms which bring together:

> *the local NHS with local authorities and others, including the voluntary sector, to set the strategic framework for improving health, tackling inequalities, and developing faster, more convenient services of a consistently high standard;*
>
> *involve all with an interest and in particular:*
>
> – *engage PCGs in the strategic planning process, ensuring that the HImP is guided by the perspective and knowledge that they are able to bring to bear, and takes proper account of locally determined needs, as well as national priorities;*
> – *enable hospital clinicians to contribute their expertise on how best to meet local needs;*

FIGURE 1.1

THE HEALTH IMPROVEMENT PROGRAMME 'CYCLE'

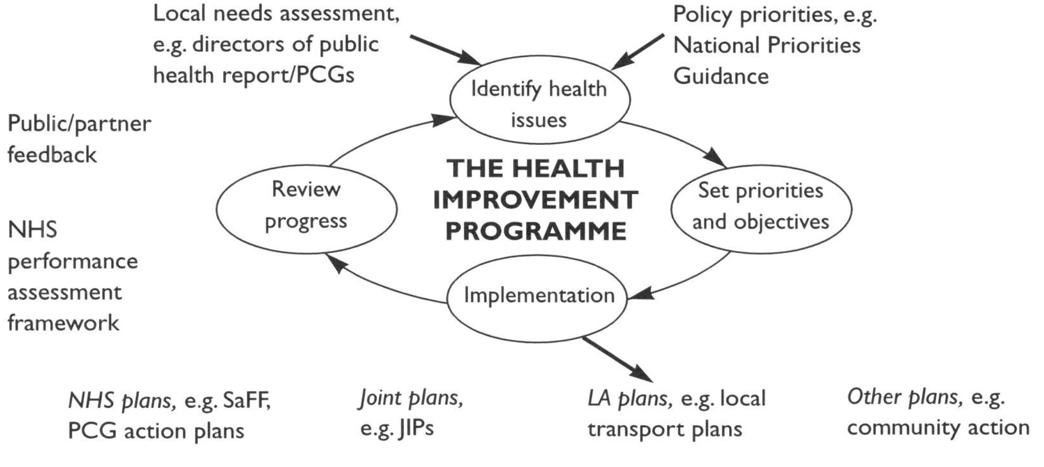

Source: HSC 1998/167 Supporting Guidance, p.2.

- *offer the opportunity for the local community and its leaders, e.g. local councillors, to influence the strategy.* (HSC 1998/167, p.4)

The way this is intended to work is set out in Figure 1.1, which sketches the intended relationships between the health improvement programme and the wider environment.

The guidance recognises that not everything can be done immediately. Nevertheless it sets out a demanding set of tasks, which are inherent in the deceptively simple Figure above. Just persuading the local health economy to work together on issues of common interest would be a substantial task – as experience of planning for annual winter crises has indicated. But on top of this, the guidance reminds health authorities of the scale of the national agenda – the introduction of national service frameworks, joint investment plans for older people (see Section 1.2) and the national targets set in *Saving Lives* (see Section 1.3), not to mention the performance measures embodied in the national performance assessment framework. While the Figure identifies these, it does not consider the Government's continuing preoccupation with the national waiting list total and other centrally managed policies, and fails to show the links between service change and the planning of capital investment. In so doing, it side-steps the awkward question of how local and national priorities will be reconciled.

COMMISSIONING

The New NHS promised an end to annual contracting and the introduction of longer-term agreements. What this was to mean in practice was originally spelt out in Circular EL (97) 39. In *Commissioning in the New NHS* (HSC 1998/198, 1 November 1998), the arrangements were spelled out in more detail, reflecting the consultations which had taken place earlier in the year.

The draft guidance attached to the Circular sets out the main features of long-term service agreements. In particular:

- *they will reflect an ongoing dialogue between clinicians, users and carers as well as managers;*
- *they will engage all those who contribute to a pathway of care, to build mutual understanding of the contributions that both primary and secondary care and, where appropriate, social care are to make, and how these can best meet patients' needs;*
- *they will include measurable targets for improvement and clear links to the performance assessment framework;*
- *they will be dynamic, incorporating incentives for improving quality and cost-effectiveness; and as part of this, they will reflect clear responsibility for risk management, ensuring activity does not get out of kilter with funding;*
- *they will form the basis for a continuing, open and co-operative relationship between the HA/PCG, NHS Trusts and Social Services to ensure that the objectives set out in the agreement are being achieved and that any difficulties are promptly resolved.* (Annex C)

The draft guidance is not specific as to how these tasks will be discharged. As noted already, variations in the scale of PCGs mean that many will not be well placed to discharge these tasks, and while the time period envisaged for the agreement – three years – is intended to allow the planning of change in delivery methods, how such planning is to be carried out and what the relationship with national frameworks should be is unclear.

Some of the tasks set out above are technically very demanding – particularly the derivation of performance measures and incentive structures. There is virtually no experience in this country of devising, implementing and monitoring the effect of these, separately or together, on clinical performance. *The New NHS* referred to the possibility of introducing incentives to clinicians responsible for delivering particular services, but so far no national advice has been issued as to how to create them.

Furthermore, the scale of many health care services is much greater than the areas for which primary care groups are responsible. In October 1998 *Commissioning in the New NHS* (HSC 1998/198) proposed that services should be subject to the new arrangements for specialised commissioning where:

i) *the planning population is significantly greater than that of a single (average-sized) health authority, because patient numbers are small, and a critical mass is required at each centre to:*

- *ensure optimum outcomes and sustain clinical competence;*
- *sustain training of specialised staff;*
- *support high quality programmes of research;*
- *ensure cost-effectiveness of provision;*
- *ensure best use of scarce resources (including expertise, high-tech equipment, donor organs).*

ii) *the service is in a fast-developing area, probably high-tech, where development and innovation need managing.*

iii) *there are high profile ethical issues (e.g. around equity of access, or high cost for small numbers of patients) on which a region-wide approach is beneficial.* (Annex A)

It went on to identify a long list of services that exhibit at least one of these characteristics (see Table 1.2).

The new NHS Modern and Dependable: primary care groups; delivering the agenda (HSC 1998/228, 8 December 1998) notes that there is a range of

TABLE 1.2

SPECIALISED SERVICES

1. Bone marrow transplant services, including PSBC transplants
2. Burns services
3. Cleft lip and palate services
4. Cystic fibrosis services
5. Gender dysphoria (includes mental health and surgery services)
6. Genetics services
7. Haemophilia services
8. Specialised services for HIV/AIDS
9. Intestinal failure services
10. Neurosciences
11. Renal replacement therapy for end-stage renal failure
12. Services for rare cancers
13. Specialised cardiology/cardiac surgery
14. Specialised maternity services
15. Specialised mental health services
16. Specialised pathology services
17. Specialised services for addictions
18. Specialised services for infectious diseases (including drug-resistant TB and viral haemorrhagic fevers)
19. Specialised services for people with learning disabilities
20. Specialised services for people with physical disabilities and chronic illness
21. Spinal injuries services
22. Tertiary services for children

Source: HSC 1999/198, Annex B.

commissioning routes:

- the health authority and the PCG working together
- each PCG working on its own
- each locality or practice working on its own, albeit within the group framework.

However, most routine, non-specialised hospital services such as A&E serve larger areas than the typical primary care group, so co-ordination will still be required to purchase them. The Circular notes that 'there is a need to balance the need to be responsive to local need and circumstances with the need to realise economies of scale, maintain standards and manage risk', but it does not indicate how that delicate balance should be found.

As the King's Fund-led national evaluation of total purchasing pilots found, sites that tried to change services such as maternity found it hard precisely because they were only part of the market the hospital served. PCGs will be larger but will still be faced with the task of co-ordinating plans for change across a number of organisations, whose priorities may differ.

As we noted last year, the role of the National Specialist Commissioning Advisory Group survived the new purchasing arrangements. This year saw only a small extension of its activities through the designation of two new services – the Kasai procedure and amyloidosis – and one new unit for paediatric liver disease.

OVERALL

The structure of the 'new NHS' is slowly emerging in terms of its formal organisation, but very little clarity has emerged during the year as to how the new institutions will develop and how they and the old institutions will work together. The general duty of co-operation imposed on the NHS – and local authorities – by the Health Act, and the many specific areas noted above where co-operation is required, are only the latest in a series of measures that successive governments have taken since the founding of the NHS to encourage the greater integration of its parts.

What has emerged, however, is that while *The New NHS* embodied elements of continuity, it has in fact subjected the whole of the NHS to a demanding programme of change. Although the scale of the changes that the Government is seeking to bring about is acknowledged – in, for example, the National Priorities Guidance issued in September 1998, which briefly sets out the Executive's view of 'how it will work' – there is no acknowledgement of what the obstacles to effective working might be.

It is not surprising therefore that doctors' representatives at, for example, the 1999 annual conference of the British Medical Association complained about the scale of the new tasks placed upon them and the speed at which change was required. To others, however, the new arrangements do seem to offer genuine scope for development at local level, which they are keen to exploit. Against the background of experiences with GP fundholding and total purchasing, the prospect would seem to be that different parts of the local NHS will develop at different speeds and in different ways. In this respect the 'new NHS' is not unlike its predecessor.

1.2 Community care

The Government has announced a vast range of new policies; their implementation may prove to be difficult.

Almost a year after its White Paper on the NHS, the Government published *Modernising Social Services*, which it described as 'the most radical overhaul of the social services system in thirty years' (PR 1998/0557, 30 November 1998). The White Paper's central argument is that social services need to:

- *seek to promote people's independence while treating them with dignity and respect at all times, and protecting their safety*
- *provide services more consistently across the country*
- *make the system more centred on service users and their families, and as convenient and straightforward as possible for people to use*. (*Modernising Social Services*, para.2.4)

As far as the first of these – the promotion of independence – is concerned, it sets out the guiding principle of adult social services in the following terms:

> *that they provide the support needed by someone to make most use of their own capacity and potential*. (*Modernising Social Services*, para.2.5)

The current pattern of care, it argues, is inappropriate, because:

> *All too often, the reverse is true, and they are regarded as services which do things for and to dependent people*. (*Modernising Social Services*, para.2.5)

The 'independence' objective and the subsequent critique of the *status quo* are little different from that accepted by the previous government when it published *Caring for People* in 1990, as the following extract shows.

> *The changes outlined in this White Paper are intended to:*
>
> - *enable people to live as normal a life as possible in their own homes or in a homely environment in the local community;*
> - *provide the right amount of care and support to help people achieve maximum possible independence and, by acquiring or reacquiring basic living skills, help them to achieve their full potential;*
> - *give people a greater individual say in how they live their lives and the services they need to help them to do so*.
>
> *Promoting choice and independence underlies all the Government's proposals*. (*Caring for People*, para.1.8)

The underlying perception, then as now, was that the way that services were provided reflected the interests of the providers themselves rather than users – and, more specifically, that too many people were being moved prematurely into residential forms of accommodation and were not being given sufficient help to remain in their own homes. Against that background, it is not surprising to find that, as we have reported in earlier Reviews, local authorities have tended to focus their resources on the most dependent people, i.e. those who might appear to be at most risk of going into institutionalised care, and have thereby reduced the total number of people to whom they provide care.

The most recent *Community Care Statistics* (Department of Health, 1997) confirm this. In 1998, there was a slight fall in the number of contact hours, but a large fall in the number of households visited. Thirty per cent of households received five or more hours (28 per cent in the previous year and 12 per cent in 1993) and 23 per cent received only one visit of less than two hours (23 and 37 per cent respectively).

The White Paper, recognising this trend, notes that:

> *... councils are tending to focus more and more on those most dependent people living in their community. For example, although there has been an increase in the overall level of domiciliary care supporting people in their own homes, that increase has been concentrated on those getting more intensive support, and the number of people receiving lower levels of support has actually dropped.* (*Modernising Social Services*, para.2.6)

But the White Paper argues that this emphasis on the most dependent is misplaced because it:

> *... means that some people who would benefit from purposeful interventions at a lower level of service, such as an occasional visit from a home help, or over a shorter period, such as training in mobility and daily living skills to help them cope with visual impairment, are not receiving any support. This increases the risk that they in turn become more likely to need much more complicated levels of support as their independence is compromised. That is good neither for the individual nor, ultimately, for the social services, the NHS and the taxpayer.* (*Modernising Social Services*, para.2.6)

King's Fund research supports the view that the faults that the Conservatives' reforms were designed to eliminate still exist. *A New Era for Community Care?: what people want from health, housing and social care services* (Farrell C, Robinson J and Fletcher P. London: King's Fund, 1999) concluded that:

> *far from promoting independent living and enabling people to live an 'ordinary life,' services often appear to reinforce dependency and social exclusion'.* (p.4)

Furthermore, *Nursing Home Placements for Older People in England and Wales: a national audit 1995–1998*, a report from St George's Department of Geriatric Medicine by the NHS Clinical Audit Unit found that four out of five residents appeared to have been receiving no care services in the community prior to admission to a nursing home – though that finding may in part reflect poor documentation. This study also found a widespread failure to provide rehabilitation services and poor medical supervision within the homes themselves. So, although some people did improve after entering them, others did not, even though they could have done so with appropriate support. *Modernising Social Services* offers no evidence of its own, however, in support of its critique of the way that resources are currently allocated; nor does it offer any advice that would help local authorities to make a more effective allocation of the resources at their disposal.

The overall objective would appear to be the same as that pursued by the previous government – the difference lies in the belief implicit in the White Paper that loss of independence can be anticipated and prevented, or at least delayed, by appropriate intervention. It does not dwell on the fate of the highly dependent if their level of support is cut so that others may be offered services that might reduce their chances of becoming highly dependent. Diversion of resources from those who are currently most dependent threatens to reduce their independence.

If this approach is to work, it must be founded on accurate identification of those at risk. Some guidance as to how authorities should approach this task is offered in *Promoting Independence: Preventative Strategies and Support for Adults* (LAC (99)14). It states that:

> *In developing their preventative strategy authorities should:*
>
> *i. attempt to move away from an emphasis on concentrating resources on people with the*

highest levels of dependency, and

ii. *look instead at how they can target interventions either*
   - *to prevent people from deteriorating to such high levels of dependency, or*
   - *to improve such people's quality of life by increasing their independence (e.g. by assisting people of working age into employment).* (LAC (99) 14, para.8)

It goes on to make a number of methodological suggestions, none of which are supported by evidence or indeed any form of factual information, as to what might work best and at what cost.

Modernising Social Services proposes three new forms of grant, which will draw on the Social Services Modernisation Fund to the tune of £750 million over three years. All are designed to encourage local authorities to develop services in line with the Government's view of where the priorities lie and one, the prevention grant, is designed to stimulate the development by local authorities of the preventative strategies envisaged in the Circular, targeting low level support for people most at risk of losing their independence.

The White Paper develops the independence theme in two other ways: first, by supporting the extension of the direct payments scheme (see *Health Care UK 1997/98*) by removing the age limit of 65; and secondly, by helping social service users gain jobs through extending The New Deal (originally focused on the young unemployed) to older workers and the disabled. While both measures are welcome, they do little to help social service authorities devise effective preventative strategies.

PARTNERSHIP

Successive Health Policy Reviews have reported evidence of the failure of health, social services and housing to work together. As noted in Section 1.1, the new direction for the NHS is based in part upon better relationships between health authorities founded on a new duty to co-operate set out in the Health Act 1999. The Act introduces a similar duty on health and local authorities:

> *In exercising their respective functions NHS bodies ... and local authorities ... shall co-operate with one another in order to secure and advance the health and welfare of the people of England and Wales.* (s.27(2))

In September 1998, prior to the publication of the Health Bill, the Government issued *Partnership in Action*, described as a consultative document 'which sets out our plans to make partnership a reality'. The paper argues that joint working is needed at three levels:

- *strategic planning: agencies need to plan jointly for the medium term, and share information about how they intend to use their resources towards the achievement of common goals;*
- *service commissioning: when securing services for their local populations, agencies need to have a common understanding of the needs they are jointly meeting, and the kind of provision likely to be most effective;*
- *service provision: regardless of how services are purchased or funded, the key objective is that the user receives a coherent integrated package of care and that they, and their families, do not face the anxiety of having to navigate a labyrinthine bureaucracy. (Partnership in Action, p.6)*

It acknowledged that 'More still needs to be done to address the boundary problems between health and social services.' But *Partnership in Action* rejected major structural change of the kind that the Health Committee of the House of Commons favoured in its report *The Relationship between Health and Social Services* (London: Stationery Office, 1999) (see Box 1.3). Instead it made three proposals to assist partnership, all of which required legislation:

- ***pooled budgets** – where health and social services put a proportion of their funds into a mutually accessible joint budget to enable* *more integrated care;*

- ***lead commissioning*** *– where one authority transfers funds to the other who will then take responsibility for purchasing both health and social care;*
- ***integrated provision*** *– where one organisation provides both health and social care.* (p.8)

The Health Act 1999 provides the necessary powers, but they are permissive, which means that it will be up to local and health authorities to decide between themselves which arrangements if any will be most helpful for their joint working.

Modernising Social Services also identifies five areas where new specific links are to be made. These include the statutory duty of partnership; the establishment of primary care groups, which are intended to work closely with social services on both planning and delivery of services and which will have social services representation on their governing bodies; and the introduction of health improvement programmes, which are also intended to involve local government and voluntary bodies. In addition, local authority chief executives are to participate in health authority meetings and there are to be joint investment plans within the health improvement programme, drawn up between health and social services to deal particularly with groups where co-ordinated services are most important.

BOX 1.3: THE HEALTH/SOCIAL CARE BOUNDARY

In December 1998 the Health Committee published a report on *The Relationship between Health and Social Services*, which welcomed the proposals in *Partnership in Action*, but found it was not radical enough:

> *... we consider that the problems of collaboration between health and social services will not be properly resolved until there is an integrated health and social care system, whether this is within the NHS, within local government or within some new, separate organisation. We acknowledge that such an integration would lead to an emphasis of the boundary between the health and social care body and other functions, for instance housing and education, but we believe it is the only sensible long-term solution to end the current confusion. Implementation of the White Paper and in particular the involvement of social services and community NHS trusts in PCGs and PCTs, provides an excellent opportunity for improved collaboration between health and social services, but falls well short of unifying the two agencies.* (para.68)

The Government response to this (Cm. 4320. London: Stationery Office, 1999) stated that:

> *The Government notes that formally integrating health and social services was not widely supported during the course of the Committee's inquiry. This lack of support for structural change was echoed during the consultation on Partnership in Action. The proposals in Partnership in Action allow for much closer ways of working including, as the Committee recognise, integrated provision and lead commissioning. These approaches will be taken forward in areas where all partners agree that they would benefit patients and service users. They will allow much greater flexibility in working across this interface than at present and provide a framework to develop working arrangements from the ground up. In addition, Primary Care Trusts will for the first time bring management of primary care and community health services together and involve social services in the governing arrangements. Primary Care Trusts will also be able to make use of the new operational flexibilities. The Government does not believe it is necessary to formally integrate health and social services.* (p.13)

To promote more effective collaboration between health and social services, the White Paper announced a partnership grant, which is intended to put:

> ... *particular emphasis on improving rehabilitation services, avoiding unnecessary admissions to hospital and other institutional care; improving discharge arrangements; and fostering good joint contingency planning to deal with emergency pressures.* (*Modernising Social Services*, p.17)

It is to be used for measures such as:

- more, and more flexible, provision of short-term intensive packages of non-residential services
- improved arrangements for health and social services to deal jointly with cases 'out of hours'
- improved multidisciplinary assessment procedures
- improved rehabilitation and recuperation arrangements
- the development of schemes for the rehabilitation of people to enable them to maintain their current employment or enter or re-enter employment
- the continuation of schemes which have been funded using 'winter pressures' money to enable these schemes to become established and integrated into mainstream services.

As the last item indicates, authorities are specifically required to address the national target set out in the National Priorities Guidance and the Department of Health's 'contract' with the Treasury, that average per capita growth in emergency hospital admissions of persons aged 75 or over should be reduced to 3 per cent (see Section 2.1).

Previous Reviews drawing on research supported by the Rowntree Foundation and the Audit Commission have pointed to the importance of housing to the achievement of the aims of community care. *Modernising Social Services* acknowledges this:

> *The Government recognises the crucial role housing has to play in community care and the need for partnership between health, housing and social services in supporting people in the community. This partnership needs to involve not only the statutory authorities but also housing providers to ensure that housing needs are identified and strategies developed to address them.* (para.6.17)

But despite this acknowledgement, the White Paper has little new to offer by way of policy initiatives. It merely notes that an interdepartmental review of funding for supported accommodation is underway and that changes are to be made to the building regulations designed to improve the accessibility of all new homes. In recognising that 'there is more to be done', it points only to the guidance already issued and the proposed long-term care charter (see Section 1.4). No proposals are made for changing the national policy framework, despite the criticisms made in the Audit Commission's report *Home Alone* of the pattern of incentives facing local authorities, which in fact encourage them to place people in residential care. *Supporting People*, the Government's proposals published in September 1998 for support services for all vulnerable people, including rough sleepers and drug users as well as frail elderly people and those with a learning disability, proposed a unification of the various funding streams including housing benefit, but these do not bear on the wide range of issues the Commission identified.

CARERS

In March 1999 the Government published *Caring about Carers: a national strategy for carers*. The approach it set out has three elements: information, support and care. It also comprises a large range of measures bearing on access to housing, work, benefits and, in the case of young carers, schooling.

In support of these measures, *Modernising Social*

Services introduced a third new grant to enhance provision of community care services to allow carers to take a break from caring by stimulating greater diversity and flexibility in provision; to encourage a greater awareness by local authorities of the need for services in their area that are more responsive to the needs of carers; and to enable carers and their organisations explicitly to be involved in work by local authorities on the appropriateness of current provision and the possibility of greater diversity. The grant is available on two conditions – that it is spent on relevant community care services and that local authorities provide a plan setting out what they intend to do and how they intend to do it. In June 1999 a Caring for Carers award was announced.

Taken together, these proposals represent a much greater commitment to the support of carers than any previous government has made. But the White Paper is permissive rather than directive, leaving the pace of implementation to be determined by the interplay of resources and local priorities.

LONG-TERM CARE

The Royal Commission on Long-term Care, *With respect to old age* reported in March 1999. It made two central recommendations:

- the costs of long-term care should be split between living costs, housing costs and personal care
- the Government should establish a National Care Commission to monitor trends, including demography and spending; ensure transparency and accountability in the system; represent the interests of consumers; and set national benchmarks now and in the future.

The Commission accepted the continuation of a health/social care dividing line but proposed that it should be shifted and that, as a result, charges for personal care would be eliminated.

> *Personal care, because it directly involves touching a person's body, incorporates issues of intimacy, personal dignity and confidentiality. Because of risks associated with poor personal care (e.g. risks of infection or skin breakdown), it is important that when the level or type of care needed becomes greater than can normally be provided at home by a relative or informal carer, careful assessment is made of how best it can be provided and by whom. It, therefore, differs qualitatively from living costs and housing costs. In recommending that personal care should be exempted from means testing, we are not recommending that this should happen on demand. Far from it, we have stressed throughout our report the importance of proper assessment of need.* (Royal Commission Report, para.6.44)

The central financial argument was that the need for long-term care was not an appropriate risk for an individual to cover and that the private sector would not do so adequately. However, in seeking to draw the line between free and means-tested care in a more logical place, the Commission committed the apparently unforgivable sin of proposing an increase in public spending by shifting the line between free and means tested so as to include personal care. It estimated that it would cost an extra £800 million to £1.2 billion, although the cost would rise over time.

As last year's Review anticipated, the Commission did not manage to achieve consensus, even within its own ranks. While the majority of the Commission plumped for an extension of the scope of free care to include all nursing as well as personal care, a minority did not, putting forward counter proposals of their own which, they argued, would make better use of limited public funds.

Not surprisingly the reaction of the Secretary of State to the Commission's report was muted:

> *The Government's response must await the outcome of that debate which I hope and expect will commence with today's publication of the Royal Commission's report.* (PN 1999/0444)

The Government made no positive steps to encourage this debate but the Select Committee, in *Long-term Care of the Elderly*, a short report published in April 1999, urged that the report should not be 'allowed to gather dust when care for older people in this country is in desperate need of a radical shake-up.' In its response, the Government did not promise a rapid action. However, in July 1999, the Court of Appeal heard a case (QBCOF99/01110/CM54) brought by a Ms Coughlan against her health authority's decision to move her out of NHS care. Ms Coughlan's case was upheld but the judgement confirmed that it was lawful for social services to provide some nursing care, albeit not of the intensity that Ms Coughlan required, in the following terms:

> *The NHS does not have sole responsibility for all nursing care. Nursing care for a chronically sick patient may be in appropriate cases provided by a local authority as a social service and that patient may be liable to meet the cost of that care according to the patient's means … Whether it is unlawful (for responsibility to be transferred from health to local authority) depends, generally, on whether the nursing Services are merely (i) incidental or ancillary to the provision of the accommodation which a local authority is under a duty to provide and (ii) of a nature which it can be expected that an authority whose primary responsibility is to provide social services can be expected to provide.* (Judgement, para.118)

The judgement was welcomed by the Secretary of State, no doubt relieved by the fact that the Court of Appeal had not decided that it was unlawful for local authorities to provide any form of nursing care. But while it clarified the position for Ms Coughlan, it still left the boundary issue far from resolved. Thus by the time the Review went to press, the situation remained just as it was before the Government came to office.

SERVICE FRAMEWORKS

We noted last year that mental health was chosen as one of the first two national service frameworks. Before that was announced, in March 1999 the Government set out its proposals for mental health services in a White Paper, *Modernising Mental Health Services*, which argues that there have been too many failures:

- *a group of service users has begun to emerge with severe mental illnesses – typically schizophrenia – who are socially isolated, difficult to engage and obviously in need of care in the long term: care in the community has often failed to deliver the treatment and support they need;*

- *families who contributed willingly to the care of people with mental illness, have found they are overburdened;*

- *inadequate systems, poor management of resources and underfunding have resulted in widespread and unacceptable variation in standards;*

- *problems of recruitment, retention and poor staff morale are commonplace, particularly in the inner cities.* (*Modernising Social Services*, para.3.2)

To remedy these deficiencies, the White Paper proposes a series of improvements including more beds, better outreach services, better access to new anti-psychotic drugs, 24-hour crisis teams, more and better trained staff, and regional commissioning teams for secure services and development teams – all to be backed by additional spending of £700 million.

In May 1999 the Government also indicated that it would take action 'to make mental health services safer' in the light of *Safer Services*, a report based on the National Confidential Inquiry into Suicide and Homicide. In PN 1999/0272, the Government states:

> *The statistics show that there is scope to prevent some of these tragic incidents. Of the cases that the Confidential Inquiry looked at – almost a quarter of suicides were known to have been in contact with mental health services in the year before death; of these, more than a quarter were known to be non-compliant with drug treatments in the month before death. 4% of all suicides (over 4000 a year) were psychiatric in-patients and around one-third of in-patient suicides occurred on the ward itself.* (p.1)

In July 1999 the Home Office and the Department of Health issued a consultation paper *Managing Dangerous People with Severe Personality Disorder: proposals for policy development*, which put forward the option of powers being introduced to retain people who might be dangerous to the public even though they had not actually committed an offence.

In March 1999 it was announced that a national service framework would be developed for the care of elderly people. The main issues to be considered were identified as:

- acute hospital care, including palliative care
- models of primary and community care
- transitions to, from and within hospital
- models of assessment and care management
- mental illness
- physical and psychological injuries caused by accidents
- stroke

The results of this work are not expected until April 2000. However, in an earlier initiative, *Better Services for Vulnerable People*, the Government required all health and local authorities to draw up joint investment plans for developing services 'to help people get the care they need while avoiding unnecessary hospital or care home admissions. This may include developing specialist rehabilitation services to help people go back home after a hospital stay or other initiatives such as dedicated discharge teams'.

The joint investment plans, according to *Better Services for Vulnerable People: maintaining the momentum*, a letter issued to chief executives on 20 August 1998, are intended:

- *to improve the ability of people to live independently through better co-ordinated local services*
- *to improve partnership working between agencies with greater transparency about current and future spending and the development of services at the health/social care interface*
- *to acknowledge issues of service quality and effectiveness and to inform agreed strategic objectives and service development priorities*
- *to produce the information necessary to support the reshaping of services across the local health and social care economy*
- *to contribute to the preparation and delivery of HImPs by putting into operation health improving strategies that span the health/social care interface.*

Joint investment plans for older people, including those with mental health problems, were to be in place by April 1999; those for other groups were to be ready a year later. Over and above the general objectives set out above, the plans are specifically intended to bear on the national target of avoiding unnecessary admissions to hospital as well as on long-term care.

REGULATION

Modernising Social Services argues that the existing regulatory arrangements suffer from three weaknesses:

- ***lack of independence** – local and health authorities have to combine responsibilities for purchasing, providing and regulating care services;*

- ***lack of coherence** – responsibilities are split between different authorities and different professional disciplines (social services professionals on the one hand, and most* *professional nurses on the other)*;

- ***lack of consistency*** – *standards vary from one area to another, creating uncertainty for both providers and service users*. (Annex A)

It therefore proposes a new system of regulation involving independent regional authorities or commissions for care standards, which will be independent statutory bodies, covering:

- residential care homes for adults
- nursing homes
- children's homes
- domiciliary social care providers
- independent fostering agencies
- residential family centres
- boarding schools.

This implies an extension of regulation to services not hitherto covered, including specifically domiciliary care. However, these proposals omit home health care services to people living in their own home, with relatives or in sheltered accommodation, which they are paying for out of their own pocket. As the King's Fund evidence to the Select Committee put it:

> *For one service provider to be regulated where another is not clearly leaves anomalies of the sort the Government appears to wish to see removed. An individual would receive regulated nursing care in a residential or nursing home but unregulated nursing care at their own home, even if the nursing tasks being carried out were identical in both settings. Further, whilst local authorities will be required to only contract with regulated domiciliary social care providers on behalf of users, the NHS will be free to contract with unregulated independent sector home healthcare providers, quite likely on behalf of the same vulnerable users*. (Report, Vol. II. Evidence, para.30, p.382)

The need for effective regulation of care homes for the elderly emerged clearly from *Older People as Consumers in Care Homes*, a report by the Office of Fair Trading issued in October 1998. Its main emphasis is on information; its central finding: 'vital information is not reaching those who need it when they need it most'. More specifically it recommends greater clarity in the initial care assessment and in the contracts between providers and residents.

In July 1999 the Health Committee of the House of Commons published its report on *The Regulation of Private and other Independent Healthcare*, which, though primarily focused on health care, took note of the need to draw the proper connections between health and social care provision. It also recommended tightening up the regulation of mental health services, where the private sector has developed a range of specialist services used largely by the NHS, and that specific links should be made between the work of the Mental Health Act Commission and that of the proposed Regional Commissions for Care Standards.

THE NEW MANAGERIALISM

Modernising Social Services affirms that 'social services need direction if they are to serve adults better'. It also makes it clear where the new direction for social services is to come from – the centre.

Over and above the wide range of initiatives briefly described above, it also sets out the 'best value' framework, already announced for local government as a whole, as it will apply to social care:

> *Best value is the key element in the Government's agenda to improve the quality of local authority services and the efficiency and economy with which they are delivered. The duty of best value – to deliver services to standards covering both cost and quality, by the most effective, economic and efficient means available – will be supported by a new Performance Management Framework*. (*Modernising Social Services*, p.9)

As this citation indicates, the new approach is to be supported by performance management. The White Paper goes on:

> *The Framework will provide a process by which a local authority can, in collaboration with its local community, question how it provides its services and how well it performs in comparison to the best performers. But best value should be seen as more than just a process, it is about a cultural change, redefining perceptions of the way local services should be delivered and the way services relate to local people.* (*Modernising Social Services*, p.9)

In February 1999, the Government issued a consultation document, *A New Approach to Social Services Performance*. For some time both the Department of Health and, as part of the Citizen's Charter initiative, the Audit Commission have published social service performance indicators. The difference between these and the new proposals lies in the way the Government intends them to be used. The Commission's indicators were intended for the general public; the Government's are intended to form part of its new management regime.

This new framework effectively puts local authorities in the position of being sub-contractors to central government, with their performance being managed by a distant, but nevertheless active, 'head office'. In the words of the consultation document:

> *The publication of the Performance Assessment Framework and the performance of individual authorities against the National Social Services Performance Indicators will provide a mechanism by which authorities are held accountable for their performance to local people and to Central Government. The performance of local social services authorities as a whole against these Performance Indicators will also provide a measure of the Government's success in delivering its programme for social care.* (*A New Approach to Social Services Performance*, para.2.12)

The question *Modernising Social Services* does not pose is: how should the head office be resourced to carry out the functions that it specifies?

OVERALL

The developments described in this Section do appear to amount to a 'radical overhaul' of the social services system – they are certainly more extensive than any previous set of policies published in so short a time. As Figure 1.2 indicates the Government has introduced a wide range of initiatives bearing on the provision of social care.

But they are perhaps better seen as 'radical incrementalism' in that the Government has aimed to work within existing administrative boundaries and retained the separation between health, social services and housing. The Government's hope is that the weaknesses stemming from that separation can be overcome by its financial innovations, the duty to co-operate and the ties that it is creating within health improvement programmes and the boards of primary care groups.

But the fundamentals remain the same and, in social policy as in market economics, the fundamentals tend to assert themselves even if in the short run new policies and events obscure them. One of those fundamentals is a lack of knowledge of what works and how individuals and their families respond to what government and others offer them, as well as to changes in their own financial circumstances. Moreover, as the Clinical Audit report cited above indicates, information about what is going on is fragmentary. While the goal of personal independence is one most would share, how to promote it more effectively is scarcely clearer than it was at the beginning of the decade.

FIGURE 1.2

NEW INITIATIVES IN SOCIAL CARE

NHS

The New NHS – Modern, Dependable

A First Class Service (National service frameworks clinical governance performance assessment framework)

Information for Health

Working Together – quality workforce for the NHS

Our Healthier Nation

With Respect to Old Age: (Royal Commission on Long-Term Care)

Modernising Health and Social Services: Joint Priorities Guidance 1999-2000 – 2001-2002

Caring About Carers: A National Strategy for Carers

Social Services Performance assessment framework

Better Government for Older People (Older people's mental health)

Health Bill (pooled budgets local commissioning service integration)

Health Improvement Programmes (HImPs)

Primary care groups (PCGs)

Joint investment plans (JIPs)

Partnership grant/prevention grant

Better Services for Vulnerable People (BSVP)

Partnership in Action: a discussion document

Winter pressures initiative

You and Your Services (long-term care charter, involving users and carers)

- Promoting Independence
- Inter-agency working
- Performance Improvement

Local Authorities

Modernising Social Services (Modernisation Fund)

Modern Local Government: In Touch with the People

Best Value (including housing, leisure and recreation)

General Social Care Council (improving training)

Social exclusion

1.3 Public health

Saving Lives: Our Healthier Nation sets out an impressive range of public health measures. Their success will depend on a number of political, financial and personal factors.

The agenda that the Government unveiled in *Saving Lives: Our Healthier Nation* was dauntingly vast. Despite its range, however, other public health issues have dominated the headlines during the past year. At the interplanetary level, astronomers reported an asteroid capable of destroying all human life heading towards the Earth, but subsequently had to admit they had lost sight of it. At an international level, while British beef started once again to be a tradeable commodity – although the Germans refused to accept it – the safety of American beef, produced with growth hormones and products containing lead compounds, became the object of an international trade row. The admission by the Belgian authorities that a deadly poison had got into the food chain led to a massive withdrawal of all food items judged to be potentially affected by it – but such is the flexibility of international trade that products banned in Belgium were imported into other countries where they were repackaged and, as a result of that process, quite legally lost their Belgian identity. Some French red wine had to be destroyed on the suspicion that it was treated with powdered cattle blood and hence risked spreading BSE. In July, there were reports that human's milk contained high concentrations of toxic chemicals.

The introduction of genetically modified (GM) foods was slowed in the UK by public and media pressure; at the international level, it was agreed at the G7 summit in June 1999 that the introduction of GM foods should proceed with caution. Within the UK, a hospital rejected the siting of a mobile phone transmitter on its roof on the grounds that the potential risks of micro radiation were too great, while evidence emerged which suggested that mobile phones were themselves a health hazard. In June 1999 the Government demanded that all trial contact lenses should be destroyed after a single use, following a statement from the Spongiform Encephalopothy Advisory Committee that suggested there was a risk – in the words of the Committee, probably a very low one – of BSE being transmitted via the eyes to the brain. Also in June the Department of Trade and Industry's Home Accident Surveillance System annual report disclosed that some 1500 products led to incidents requiring hospital treatment; happily, it did not conclude that they should all be banned. In July, there were reports that personal computers were the cause of a wide range of illnesses. Finally, scientific reports continued to appear that suggested a link between MMR vaccination and the development of autism and Crohn's disease. Because of the Government's commitment to the vaccination programme, the last of these received a rapid response. At the Chief Medical Officer's request, the Medical Research Council held a seminar involving a wide range of experts; the findings of the Royal Free Hospital group were reviewed and it was concluded that their evidence did not undermine the use of MMR. In June 1999, the deputy Chief Medical Officer, Jeremy Metters, and the Chairman of the Committee of Safety of Medicines, Professor Breckenridge, issued an 'urgent communication' drawing all doctors' attention to two reports that had found no such link. But these reports themselves were subject to strong criticism, despite their appearance in prestigious medical journals.

In July 1999 the Government's published its public health White Paper *Saving Lives: Our*

Healthier Nation, which sets out a wide range of measures bearing on two main goals:

- *to improve the health of the population as a whole by increasing the length of people's lives and the number of years people spend free from illness; and*
- *to improve the health of the worst off in society and to narrow the health gap.* (*Saving Lives: Our Healthier Nation, p.4)*

As far as the first is concerned, the White Paper sets four 'tough and challenging' targets to be achieved by 2010. These bear on reduction in mortality rather than freedom from illness:

- *cancer: to reduce the death rate in people under 75 by at least a fifth;*
- *coronary heart disease and stroke: to reduce the death rate in people under 75 by at least two-fifths;*
- *accidents: to reduce the death rate by at least a fifth and serious injury by at least a tenth;*
- *mental illness: to reduce the death rate from suicide and undetermined injury by at least a fifth.* (*Saving Lives: Our Healthier Nation*, p.1)

Following last year's Green Paper, the White Paper proposes a partnership between 'people, communities and Government'. We look at each of these elements in turn.

The White Paper sets out three policy strands for individuals, in what it terms the Healthy Citizens programme: NHS Direct (which we look at in the following Section); 'health skills', which includes training for young people as part of the Healthy Schools programme (see Box 1.4); and 'expert patients', targeted mainly at those with chronic illness.

The Chief Medical Officer is to set up a task force to design an Expert Patients programme to:

> *address the needs of the very many people in this country with a chronic disease or disability, who amount to one-in-three of the total population. The Task Force will look at the role which those affected can themselves play as experts in managing their chronic disease. It will set out the relationship between such programmes and the support which people require from the NHS. It will design a pilot programme and provide advice on what needs to be done to make services for people with chronic disease a central part of the NHS.* (*Saving Lives: Our Healthier Nation*, p.15)

This programme is designed to support those who are already keen to take more responsibility for their health. But not everyone is, and while stressing the role of individuals in safeguarding and promoting their own health, the White Paper does not face head-on some of the uncomfortable facts that current monitoring of personal behaviour reveals. The results of the annual Health Survey for England 1997 provided modest encouragement for the Government's reliance on personal responsibility. For example, the proportions of men and women reporting that they currently smoked cigarettes (29 per cent of men and 27 per cent of women) were broadly unchanged from 1993.

Seventeen per cent of men and almost 20 per cent of women were classified as obese – this compares to 13 per cent of men and 16 per cent of women in 1993. And although there was little change from 1993 in the percentage of men who reported drinking over 21 units of alcohol per week, there was an increase in the proportion of women who reported drinking more than 14 units per week – from 13 per cent in 1993 to 16 per cent in 1997. Furthermore, 36 per cent of young men and 14 per cent of young women aged 16–24 reported drinking, at least once a week, more than twice the daily amount advised as sensible.

The Government had already published a White Paper, *Smoking Kills*, in December 1998 and committed itself to a 5 per cent increase in real terms in taxation. *Smoking Kills* sets out a series of further measures designed to reduce smoking, including:

- ending tobacco advertising
- changing attitudes through public education programmes
- curtailing tobacco smuggling, the incentives for which will increase as UK tax rises
- carrying out research into the safety of nicotine replacement therapy and the effectiveness of other interventions to reduce smoking
- clean air and passive smoking – no new compulsory measures are envisaged but a number of voluntary measures including a code of practice are proposed
- support for anti-smoking measures world-wide.

The White Paper concludes with a list of all the action the Government is taking or trying to take. Wisely, it does not profess to be able to estimate their individual or total impact, but nevertheless three aims and their associated targets are set out:

> *Aim: to halt the rise in children smoking*
> *Target: to reduce smoking among children from 13% to 9% or less by the year 2010; with a fall to 11% by the year 2005.*
>
> *Aim: to establish a new downward trend in adult smoking rates in all social classes*
> *Target: to reduce adult smoking in all social classes so that the overall rate falls from 28% to 24% or less by the year 2010; with a fall to 26% by the year 2005.*
>
> *Aim: to improve the health of expectant mothers and their families*
> *Target: to reduce the percentage of women who smoke during pregnancy from 23% to 15% by the year 2010; with a fall to 18% by the year 2005.*
> (*Smoking Kills*, pp.82–84)

Smoking cessation guidelines were published in January 1998. In May 1999 *Helping Smokers Stop* (PN 1999/0276), a guide to NHS professionals was launched. At the same time the Secretary of State announced that £60 million would be allocated to smoking cessation services over three years, £10 million of that was allocated to Health Action Zones. In June the draft Tobacco (Prohibition of Advertising and Promotion) Regulations 1999 were published, containing provisions for implementing the EU directive on tobacco advertising.

The Government did not issue a White Paper on obesity. But in March 1999 Tessa Jowell, the Minister for Public Health, announced what she termed a wide-ranging plan of action, which included the Healthy Schools programme (see Box 1.4) and healthy living centres. As she acknowledged, these would not 'turn round or even halt the inexorable rise in the levels of obesity overnight. But [the measures] will make a difference in the long term' (PR 1999/0192). In contrast to the policy on smoking, none of the measures bear on producers; the Government is relying entirely on 'personal responsibility'.

The Government's approach in other areas of personal behaviour remains to be clarified. *Our Healthier Nation* promised a national strategy on alcohol misuse but it had not appeared by the time this Review was completed. In March 1999, Tessa Jowell announced the 'first ever Government strategy on sexual health' with the objectives of:

> - *improving access to services, with particular consideration of the possible benefits of integrating services for family planning and sexually transmitted diseases;*
> - *spreading good practice in service delivery, including developing stronger links between health services, families and schools; developing programmes of professional training in sexual health to move away from a compartmentalised approach;*
> - *adding value to public health campaigns by adopting a broader sexual health focus and encouraging a more mature attitude to sex.*
>
> (Department of Health 1999/0166, 23 March 1999)

BOX 1.4: SOME NEW INITIATIVES

New programmes proliferate. Here are a few:

Young and Active – the title of a report from the Health Education Authority promoting up to an hour a day of physical activity for young people.

Healthy Workplace – a broad-based initiative which aims to ensure that:

- *there is an organisational culture that actively promotes a healthy workforce, and recognises the benefits of better health for the business prospects of the organisation;*
- *there are management practices, including work design, that recognise and value the contribution of the individual to the workplace and their health needs and limitations; and*
- *there is health and safety management arrangements that minimise exposure to risk and maximise control of risk and includes access to occupational health advice and support*

Healthy Schools programme – a joint programme between health and local authorities and involving parents, children and schools to help to improve the health of both pupils and teachers. It includes:

- *a Wired for Health website – the first stage provides information for teachers on health issues, it will be developed to include information for pupils tailored to their ages;*
- *A Healthy Teacher Focus to address occupational health issues for staff; and*
- *cooks' academies in schools to improve knowledge about nutrition and develop cooking skills.*

Safer Travel to School – a joint initiative between the Department of Health and the Department of the Environment, Transport and the Regions to co-ordinate money being spent on school transport and to look at alternatives: this includes the *Safe and Sound Challenge*, which aims to increase the number of children and young people who walk or cycle to school safely through innovative travel schemes.

Sure Start is a joint Department for Education and Employment and Department of Health programme targeted at children under four and their families in areas of need. The aim is to have 250 programmes in place in England by the end of 2002. It will 'improve opportunities for all families with young children in the area' and 'In Whitehall and at regional level, cultural change and better co-ordination will underpin local efforts'.

Source: *Target*, Issue 33, March 1999.

In July, it was announced that Professor Michael Adler would lead the development of the strategy.

The Government had already published in April 1998 a White Paper, *Tackling Drugs to Build a Better Britain*, which detailed its approach to the drugs problem and its ten-year strategy for tackling drugs misuse. Attached to the White Paper was a report of the UK Anti-Drugs Co-ordinator, Keith Hellawell, which argued that:

resources for drug-specific activities should receive priority within health authorities' budgets, and on the basis of partnership work wherever appropriate. Health authorities should be required to deliver this strategy through the NHS Priorities and Planning Guidance. The development of the new NHS and Public Health White Papers should be used to ensure that health authorities give adequate provision to meeting the aims of the strategy through central guidance. Health authorities will be expected to include anti-drugs measures in their Health Improvement Programme. (The United Kingdom Anti-Drugs Co-ordinator, *First Annual Report & National Plan*. Cabinet Office, 1999, p.2)

In his annual report for 1998/99 Mr Hellawell was able to record 'good progress' in implementing the strategy set out a year earlier. That progress however was administrative in nature, including international and cabinet level co-ordinating committees, partnerships with the private sector and local drug action teams – the main mechanism for delivering the strategy on the ground. For the first time the NHS Priorities and Planning Guidance contained a reference to drugs services in relation to a reorganised grants programme to local authorities: health authorities were required to include anti-drugs measures in their health improvement programmes.

The key targets are to:

- reduce the proportion of those under 25 taking illegal drugs
- reducing repeat offending
- increase drug treatment programmes
- reduce access to drugs among 5- to 16-year-olds

Here, as with smoking, a wide range of measures is being introduced so as to effect not only the choices made by an individual, but the context – in this case the price and availability of drugs – within which they make those choices.

GOVERNMENT

Saving Lives: Our Healthier Nation notes the wide range of measures the Government has introduced which bear on health but which are the responsibility of other departments, such as the Treasury, the Department of Trade and Industry and the Department of Education and Employment and others. These include the New Deal, which is being extended from young to older workers and the disabled; more extensive child care; and increases in child benefit, the minimum wage and tax credits for low earners.

Within the traditional field of health care, the White Paper announces the Government's intention to establish a Health Development Agency, the aims of which will include:

- *maintaining an up-to-date map of the evidence base for public health and health improvement*
- *commissioning such research and evaluation as is necessary to support and strengthen the evidence base in areas where action programmes are required to improve health and tackle inequality, within an agreed framework governed by the Secretary of State's overall research strategy for health*
- *in the light of the evidence, advising on the setting of standards for public health and health promotion practice, and on the implementation of those standards by a range of organisations at national and local level*
- *in particular, providing advice on targeting health promotion most effectively on the worst off and narrowing the health gap*
- *through regular bulletins, guidance and advice, disseminating information on effectiveness and good practice in an authoritative, timely and effective manner to those working in the public health/health promotion field*
- *commissioning and carrying out evidence-based national health promotion programmes and campaigns which are integrated with the Department of Health's overall communications strategy and linked with regional and local activity*
- *advising on the capacity and capability of the public health workforce to deliver Ministers' strategy in these areas to the agreed standards, and on the education and training needs of the workforce, ensuring throughout that such advice is informed by research evidence and the appropriate quality standards*. (*Saving Lives: Our Healthier Nation*, p.2)

The White Paper also reveals the Government's plans to establish public health observatories in each NHS region. Their tasks will be:

- *monitoring health and disease trends and highlighting areas for action*
- *identifying gaps in health information*
- *advising on methods for health and health inequality impact assessments*
- *drawing together information from different sources on new ways to improve health*
- *carrying out projects to highlight particular health issues*
- *evaluating progress by local agencies in improving health and cutting inequality*
- *looking ahead to give early warning of future public health problems*. (*Saving Lives: Our Healthier Nation*, para.11.30)

It also proposes a Public Health Development Fund – worth at least £96 million over three years.

COMMUNITIES

At a local level, as at the national, many of the key levers lie with local authorities and other local agencies. *Saving Lives: Our Healthier Nation* affirms the role of education, housing, environment and policing, and, in respect of all major new Government policies, a new requirement is to be imposed: that they should be assessed for their impact on health. In the words of the White Paper:

> *Local decision-makers must think about the effect which their policies may have on health and in particular how they can reduce health inequality. In most cases this will require a change in the way that health authorities, local authorities and other local agencies see their role … An important part of this role will be to encourage all local agencies to make local health impact assessment when planning investment in, for example, amenities, buildings or local communities and in the location of services*. (*Saving Lives: Our Healthier Nation*, p.56, para.4.47)

As noted in Section 1.1, primary care groups have, as one of their three main activities, the role of improving the health of their communities. Guidance issued in *The new NHS Modern and Dependable: primary care groups; delivering the agenda* (HSC 1998/228, 8 December 1998) suggests that this might include:

- *ensuring those in greatest need are given special attention by, for example, working with Local Authorities and other agencies to help drug and alcohol misusers so that they are in a position to gain employment and face up to their addiction problems*
- *working with the local housing department to reduce falls in the elderly or with local schools to reduce smoking and drug use*
- *using community development approaches to improve the health of people who have difficulties accessing health care in some housing estates*
- *making services more responsive to needs such as ensuring better services for vulnerable people such as older people or children in care*
- *providing, in their one to one consultations with patients, health promotion and prevention interventions (e.g. smoking cessation and lifestyle advice) which can be extended by working to develop other local service initiatives such as healthy living centres*. (p.9, para.13)

How this challenging agenda should be tackled, however, remains to be determined.

We noted last year the introduction of Health Action Zones. In January 1999 the Government indicated that it was allocating £290 million over three years to first- and second-wave Zones.

Whether the Zones are effective is the subject of a national evaluation led by the Personal Social Services Research Unit at the University of Kent at Canterbury.

HEALTHY LIVING CENTRES

In January 1999, *Healthy Living Centres* (HSC 1999/008) set out the framework for the development of the centres. There are three key elements:

- *an opportunity to mobilise community*

activity in improving health and reducing inequalities;

- *a focus for bringing together health promotion in its widest sense across a broad range of interests which do not necessarily have a tradition of working together;*
- *the potential to improve access to mainstream services for those who for whatever reason do not currently use them, or to provide a better alternative to mainstream primary care.* (p.3)

As this brief extract makes clear, proposals are intended to emerge from local communities of people rather than, as with Health Action Zones, local organisations. The guidance allows up to two years for applications to be put together, thereby allowing time for local informal organisations to develop.

HEALTH INEQUALITIES

One of the central themes of *Saving Lives: Our Healthier Nation* was the Government's aim of reducing health inequalities. In November 1998 the report of the independent inquiry in health inequalities, chaired by Sir Donald Acheson, was published. This made a vast number of policy recommendations covering most fields of Government policy and a small number of general recommendations bearing on

TABLE 1.3

HEALTH ACTION ZONES

	Population
Wave 1	
Tyne and Wear	1,100,000
Manchester, Salford and Trafford	880,000
South Yorkshire Coal fields communities of Barnsley, Doncaster and Rotherham	770,000
Lambeth, Southwark and Lewisham	730,000
East London and City	580,000
Bradford	470,000
North Cumbria	320,000
Northumberland	310,000
Sandwell	300,000
Plymouth	260,000
Luton	180,000
Wave 2	
Merseyside	1,400,000
Leeds	727,000
Nottingham	640,000
Hull and East Riding	575,000
Tees	558,000
Sheffield	530,000
Cornwall and Isles of Scilly	483,000
North Staffordshire	471,000
Bury and Rochdale	389,000
Camden and Islington	365,000
Wakefield	317,000
Leicester City	295,000
Walsall	263,000
Brent	248,000
Wolverhampton	244,000

Government policy as a whole. Two of the latter were directed at better data and better monitoring mechanisms bearing on trends in inequalities and the impact of policies. A third point recommended the use of health impact assessment, which was proposed in the White Paper. As far as health services are concerned, the report recommended a focus on inequalities among women of childbearing age, expectant mothers and young children. The report identifies several further areas for action within the NHS, most of which bear on equity of access and are considered in Section 2.2.

The Government response was published at the same time as *Saving Lives. Reducing Health Inequalities: an action report*, takes each of Sir Donald's recommendations, many of which bear on the wider economic and social environment, and indicates how the Government has responded. It correctly claims that the actions set out represent 'the most comprehensive programme of work to tackle health inequalities ever undertaken in this country', but it acknowledges that:

> *A number of the policies and interventions set out in this report are at an early stage or are still being developed. Inevitably it will take some time before the full effects are felt in terms of reducing the inequalities in health that have developed over a number of years* (para.1.6)

Against this background it is perhaps not surprising that the Government did not commit itself to any specific target reductions in inequalities, leaving these to local action and health improvement plans in particular.

MONITORING PROGRESS

Recognising the long lead-time for the targets it sets, *Saving Lives: Our Healthier Nation* proposes that 2005 should be an interim 'milestone', and that every three years there will be a review of changes in:

- expectations of life
- healthy life expectancy
- health inequality.

At local level, NHS bodies are to be held to account through the new performance assessment framework for public health as well as service achievements:

> *We want the achievements of results in delivering Saving Lives: Our Healthier Nation to matter as much to local agencies as hitting the targets in the other important programmes they deliver. A health organisation should take as much pride in reaching the targets set out here as in achieving its targets on waiting lists and times. The goals in this White Paper must be as rigorously pursued by performance managers as any other targets.* (*Saving Lives: Our Healthier Nation*, para.11.46)

The White Paper does not explain what will happen if the targets prove, because of resource constraints, to be incompatible.

SCREENING

The failures of the two main screening services, those for breast and cervical cancer, have been reported in earlier Reviews and, as noted last year, the Government announced plans to overhaul their management. In March 1999 the Government responded to the Public Accounts Committee's criticisms by restating its commitment to ensuring that target coverage levels are attained and its intention to ensure that the screening system itself works well. The Government returned to the theme in *Challenging Cancer*, the statement on cancer services published in May 1999 to coincide with a 'cancer summit' hosted by the Prime Minister and presented as part of the manifesto commitment to 'making cancer a top priority'.

Challenging Cancer acknowledges that:

> *We have screening programmes for breast and cervical cancer but they have not all been well organised in the past – the services they provide have not always been of a consistently high quality. And too many women from ethnic*

minority groups or deprived inner city areas do not respond to invitations for screening. (Department of Health, 1999, p.10)

Over and above the reorganisation to the screening services, the statement indicates that all health authorities should achieve the national cervical screening target of screening 80 per cent of eligible women by 2002. Thirteen health authorities that are not meeting this target have new action plans to do so. It should be added that £6 million is being spent over the

BOX 1.5: THE HEALTH OF THE NATION

In *The Health of the Nation – a policy assessed*, one of the few systematic assessments of previous policy initiatives commissioned by the Department of Health, a review team comprising the Nuffield Institute for Health at Leeds, the Welsh Institute for Health and Social Care and the London School of Hygiene and Tropical Medicine concluded that although the initiative had been widely welcomed, it had largely failed:

Its impact on policy documents peaked as early as 1993 and, by 1997, its impact on local policymaking was negligible.

At the most general level, this failure was attributed to the identification of the initiative with the Department of Health, whereas its successful implementation required contributions from and co-ordination with local government and other central government departments. But even within the NHS itself, it was pushed aside by other priorities, particularly waiting lists and balancing the books. As a result, it:

... did not change significantly the perspective and behaviour of health authorities and did not fundamentally alter the context within which dialogue between health authorities and other partners took place. (para.2.4)

It goes on to say that although the initiative had provided a framework within which the commissioning role was to be judged:

Where attempts were made to drive progress via the contracting process, the results were minimal. The impact upon Trust and primary care teams' performance was slight. (para.2.7)

And:

The Health of the Nation *did not seriously impact upon general practitioners either as commissioners or providers.*

These findings, amplified further in the report, led the team to a large number of broad conclusions about what had to be done if the successor policies were to have a greater impact:

Greater success is likely with integrated central leadership and committed local ownership.
Building and sustaining local intersectoral partnerships and alliances will be important.
Developing the evidence base for both target setting and other implementation activities should be a key priority.
Without the requirement for substantial performance management, particularly at local level, a new public health programme's chances of success will be reduced significantly. (pp.3–4)

Source: *The Health of the Nation: a policy assessed*. London: Stationery Office, 1998.

next two years on two pilot studies to see if colorectal cancer screening is feasible, and that the case for prostate screening is being kept under review.

We noted above the concerns that the Government had addressed about the MMR vaccine. Data for 1997/98 (NHS Immunisation Statistics, England 1997/98) showed that take-up of the combined vaccine fell slightly over the previous year and remained below the level achieved in 1992/93. All other courses of immunisation showed an increase over the previous year.

RISK

The evident reluctance of many people to desist from activities that pose risks to their health should be noted. *Saving Lives* argues that:

> *... it is the role of the Government to provide information about risk. But in most cases it is for the individual to decide whether to take the risk. And there is also a balance between risk and personal freedom. Some people enjoy pursuing outdoor sports which others would consider too dangerous to undertake. As long as people are aware of the risk which they are taking, it is their decision whether to put themselves at risk.* (para.3.25)

The White Paper goes on:

> *We are currently reviewing our approach to risk and its communication. A series of seminars have involved key Ministers, the Better Regulation Task Force, senior officials, scientists, professionals, consumer representatives and journalists. The Task Force plans to make a series of recommendations as a result of these consultations.* (para.3.20)

The need for such a policy is evident from some of the events of the year. As the examples cited at the start of this Section indicate, the public is bombarded with what purports to be information about risks to health – as well as the benefits of this or that food product – some of which may be false and some of which may be accurate. Much is disregarded in part because it is not believed. As the BMA acknowledges in its May 1999 report on GM foods, *The Impact of Genetic Modification on Agriculture, Food and Health*, the public trusts neither governments nor experts – in part perhaps because of the BSE crisis and in part because of the competing claims with which it is faced.

Furthermore, the language of risk is generally inappropriate. Risks can only be assessed where activities are common and well understood; where they are not, as with GM foods, the public and governments alike are faced with uncertainty. As the report from the Chief Scientist and the Chief Medical Officer indicates, 'nothing can be absolutely certain' in a field of new technology and scientific advance. How then can change be justified when the risks are unknown?

The BMA statement argued that there should be an open-ended moratorium on commercial GM planting until there is a 'scientific consensus' on safety. The BMA stated that, 'Once the GM genie is out of the bottle, the impact on the environment is likely to be irreversible.' It therefore proposes that:

> *The precautionary principle should be applied in developing modified crops or foodstuffs, as we cannot at present know whether there are any serious risks to the environment or to human health involved in producing GM crops or consuming GM food products.* (*The Impact of Genetic Modification on Agriculture, Food and Health*, p.12)

This defers but does not eliminate the difficulty. All change involves uncertainty and hence the acceptance of some unquantified risk to health, as the statement by the Government's Chief Scientist and Chief Medical Officer, cited in Box 1.6, acknowledges. Unfortunately that statement does not offer a criterion for deciding how, if at all, to proceed. The SEAC statement cited at the beginning of this Section went on to say that '...the Committee felt strongly that the

BOX 1.6: HEALTH IMPLICATIONS OF GENETICALLY MODIFIED FOODS

The Government's Chief Scientist, Sir Robert May, and the Chief Medical Officer, Professor Liam Donaldson, issued a statement in May 1999 from which the following is extracted:

> *We have considered the processes used in genetic modification in relation to events occurring in nature and in conventional plant breeding and we conclude that there is no current evidence to suggest that the process of genetic modification is inherently harmful. Many of the issues raised by foods produced using genetic modification are equally applicable to foods produced by conventional means. We are reassured by the precautionary nature and rigour of the current procedures used to assess the safety of individual GM foods.*
>
> *Nevertheless, nothing can be absolutely certain in a field of rapid scientific and technological development. Genetic modification is a young science and there is a need to keep a close watch on developments and to continue to fund research to improve scientific understanding in this area. We welcome the recent moves to improve the openness of the regulatory procedures to public scrutiny and would encourage further such moves to help to inform public debate on the issues relating to the health implications of GM foods.* (para.83, pp.17–18)

Source: www.doh.gov.uk/gmfood.htm

Department of Health should encourage opticians to adopt, as a matter of best practice, the single use of trial lenses followed by safe disposal.' Some might think that an excessive application of the precautionary principle. But if it is appropriate, how is it to be squared with the risks arising from GM foods?

Furthermore, individuals, however well informed, cannot make sensible choices as consumers if they cannot avoid the risks concerned; this is the case with the risks that GM foods may indirectly give rise to via their impact on wildlife and other crops. The only recourse of individuals in this case is political or even direct action.

OVERALL

The Government can rightly claim that its public health White Paper represents a major advance on the previous government's *The Health of the Nation* initiative. As *Saving Lives: Our Healthier Nation* recognises, its proposals will only work if the NHS has available to it the requisite range of skills and knowledge. As far as knowledge is concerned, the White Paper makes proposals that we note in Section 1.5 below. As for skills, *Saving Lives* announced the intention to develop a Public Health Workforce National Development Plan, designed to 'unlock the potential of the entire public health workforce'.

But the obstacles that hindered the progress of *The Health of the Nation* have not disappeared and, indeed, some have become greater. Not only do individuals obstinately continue to pursue unhealthy lifestyles, the Government itself has not fully learned the lessons of that earlier initiative – that immediate service and financial pressures will push other issues to the side, particularly when they are also the object of 'performance management'. That said, the range of measures the Government has undertaken to implement is impressively wide. And even though the targets may be few in numbers, whether progress has been made – for whatever reason – will become abundantly clear.

1.4 Serving the consumer

The policy emphasis has shifted from modifying existing services to developing new ones.

The original stimulus to the introduction of the Patient's Charter was the perception that, across the public sector as a whole, services were not responsive to users. Rather, provider power ruled. The Charter set standards which providers should attain, while the publication of the results – in principle at least – gave users the information to exercise an informed choice of where to seek treatment. In practice, such informed choice was limited, so the main burden of making the service user responsive lay largely with the Charter's impact on providers. There were signs, with the patient–partnership initiative, of a different approach developing towards the end of the Conservatives' period of office. But when Labour came to office, the Charter remained the most obvious embodiment of Government commitment to the user, as opposed to the provider, interest. As we record below, the Government has now moved on to more substantive measures.

THE PATIENT'S CHARTER

The Labour Party's election manifesto promised a review of the Patient's Charter as well as a reduction in the numbers waiting for elective hospital treatment by 100,000. The first of these commitments proved easier to fulfil than the second. In November 1998, Greg Dyke, now Director-General of the BBC, published his (personal) proposals for a new form of an NHS Charter to replace the existing Patient's Charter. In his view, the aims of a new charter should be:

- *to explain to the patients the standards of care they can expect from the NHS and for this to be effectively monitored*
- *to give the patient information to enable her or him to become a partner in determining the type of care and treatment they receive*
- *to empower patients to be more explicit about their views of the service they receive including a clear explanation of means of redress*
- *to improve levels of communication throughout the NHS.* (*Report on the New NHS Charter. Department of Health*, p.5)

Against this anodyne background, he argued for a different approach. His central criticism is that:

> *A single national Charter covering all parts of the NHS is a laudable aim but, given the scale and diverse nature of the NHS, is likely to be another paper exercise.* (p.5)

He therefore proposed that the emphasis should instead be shifted to a local approach, embodying three distinct elements:

> *An NHS Value Statement*
> *There should be a clear set of values for the NHS which set out the guiding principles underpinning the service – principles which need to gain the support of both staff and patients alike.*
>
> *The Development of Local Charters*
> *Instead of a single national Charter there should be local Charters throughout the NHS ... The Charters will be largely, but not exclusively, based on locally driven priorities thus recognising the local nature of the NHS.*
>
> *Disease Specific User Guides*
> *... there should be a series of disease specific user guides produced with the aim of helping the patient understand and, more importantly, use this new comparative clinical information. The overall aim of these guides is to enable the*

patients to become more active partners in their treatment and care. (pp.5–6)

The national level approach is not rejected entirely but, Dyke argues, it should be restricted to a number of key areas, such as maximum waiting times, which would be mainly drawn from the existing Charter and included in the new local charters unless it can be demonstrated that they are not relevant to that particular part of the NHS. Dyke suggests that local charters should be piloted before their general introduction. The Government had not responded to the report by this time this Review went to press, but the third of his suggestions is close to the proposals we note below for developing NHS Direct.

As noted last year, and as a separate initiative, the Government announced that a charter for long-term care would be drawn up. The King's Fund research commissioned to support its development found, echoing Dyke's conclusions, that there was considerable cynicism about the value of charters. It concluded that any long-term care charter should address three areas:

- *the current political and social climate, recognising people's experiences of service cut-backs and their desire to see better value from current resources;*
- *the aspirations of disabled people to lead an 'ordinary life' and their common experiences of disadvantage, discrimination and social exclusion;*
- *the need for a distinctive cultural shift in community care so that services adopt a 'can do' approach.* (Farrell C, Robinson J and Fletcher P. A *New Era for Community Care?* London: King's Fund, 1999, p.3)

BOX 1.7: THE PATIENT'S CHARTER – DYKE'S CRITICISMS

- *Its potential for success hinged upon staff within the NHS owning the concept and supporting its implementation. The adoption of a top down approach meant the Charter achieved neither.*
- *The original Charter imposed national process targets upon what are fundamentally local organisations – it failed to recognise that NHS organisations are driven primarily by local needs and, as such, adapt their processes to meet these needs. I think it has to be acknowledged that there is a limit to what nationally driven targets can achieve, particularly in the areas of staff and service.*
- *The existing Charter standards concentrated disproportionately on hospitals and largely ignored the main interface between the patient and the NHS – the GP and other primary care areas. Although GPs were encouraged to develop their own practice Charters, and a large number did so, there was no monitoring of the quality or effectiveness of these Charters and little evidence that they made an impact.*

Source: *Report on the New NHS Charter.* Department of Health, p.10.

BOX 1.8: WHAT PEOPLE WANT FROM HEALTH, HOUSING AND SOCIAL CARE SERVICES

Ordinary lives

People with long-term illness or disability wanted to be able to lead an 'ordinary life'. Issues they regarded as important ingredients of independent living included:

- *choice* about where to live, about how to spend their days and about the kinds of services that are on offer
- *having a say* in their own treatment, care and support, and in the type and timing of services provided for individuals and for local populations
- *support* in getting out and about, meeting people, taking part in social activities and dealing with the practicalities of running a home
- *safety* and security in the home and in the neighbourhood.

Services

The main concerns centred on obtaining appropriate provision when needed and having ways of co-ordinating services to ensure ease of access and continuity of care. Issues included:

- *responsiveness and flexibility* in the service system as a whole, leading to timely assessments and appointments and to provision that fits individual circumstances and requirements
- *quality* relating to standards of workmanship when installing and maintaining aids and equipment and to basic and specialist skills among care staff and medical practitioners
- *service integration* where workers co-ordinate provision for individuals, where there is a single point of access to a range of services and where agencies work together to plan and deliver services.

Communication

Information was seen as the key to the provision of good services, and the way people with disabilities are treated by professionals and the public at large can make all the difference between feeling respected or rejected as an equal citizen. Issues included:

- *information* about health and treatment, about social services' eligibility criteria, assessments, complaints procedures and help available, and about housing options
- *access* to houses, public buildings and other aspects of the built environment facilitate participation in community life, and the capacity to take advantage of community services. Poor telephone and reception services, combined with complex forms used when applying for help can create unnecessary barriers to services
- *attitudes* among some professionals are experienced by disabled people as discriminatory, patronising and demeaning.

Source: Farrell C, Robinson J and Fletcher P. A *New Era for Community Care?* London: King's Fund, 1999, p.2.

In 1999, the Government published *You and Your Services* (www.doh.gov.uk/ltchart.htm), a consultation draft for the long-term care charter, which was defined in terms of 'people needing on-going support or care' and hence including people of all ages. The draft aims to set out 'the type of response which you can expect' in six areas:

- finding out about services
- understanding your needs
- the right place to live
- looking after your health
- dignity and autonomy/keeping independent
- helping carers to care.

In line with the recommendations of the Dyke report, it embodies a statement of values and also proposes the development of local charters running across health and local authority services. The consultation period concluded in August 1999.

Over much of the year, the Government appeared to be on track to fulfil its second pre-election target of cutting the numbers waiting for elective care. Between May 1997 and March 1999, the numbers recorded as waiting fell rapidly to a level lower than the Government had inherited. However, between April and May 1999 numbers rose slightly, leaving the total at 1,096,100. Moreover, the numbers waiting for over the target times for an out-patient consultation also rose.

In announcing the figures in June, the Secretary of State suggested that 'seasonal breaks in the NHS after a hard-working winter' and maintenance work on operating theatres were responsible for the rise. But:

> *we promised that by the end of this Parliament we would reduce waiting lists to 100,000 lower than the figure that we inherited. Waiting lists are already 65,000 lower and we will deliver our promises this year.* (PR 1999/0332)

While the April figures represent a setback for the Government (in its view a temporary one), it could claim success in virtually eliminating the longest waits – those over 12 months. But the increase in the numbers waiting for an out-patient appointment for over 13 weeks suggested that success in reducing the numbers waiting for admission had been achieved only by making people wait at an earlier stage in the process of gaining access to treatment.

Apart from the maximum waiting levels, the Government has not set targets for admission dates across elective care as a whole. However, in *The New NHS* the Government announced its intention to introduce a new requirement in relation to breast cancer, specifying a two-week target time between referral and consultation:

> *Everyone with suspected cancer will be able to see a specialist within two weeks of their GP deciding they need to be seen urgently and requesting an appointment.* (*The New NHS*, p.7, para.1.13)

In *Breast Cancer Waiting Times: achieving the two week target* (HSC 1998/242, 22 December 1998), the Government set out what should be done to achieve the new target. The Circular notes that:

> *2 ... Preliminary analysis of this pre-new NHS data shows that over 70% of patients referred urgently and diagnosed with breast cancer had been seen within the two weeks timescale ... Regional summaries indicate that the majority of NHS Trusts now have an average wait for urgent suspected breast cancer appointments of less than two weeks.* (HSC 1998/242, p.3)

It goes on:

> *3. The responsibility for meeting the two week target is shared between GPs and NHS Trusts. If a GP decides that a patient with suspected breast cancer needs to be seen urgently, they should reflect that urgency by ensuring that the NHS Trust receives the referral* ***within 24 hours of making that decision****, by using telephone, fax or other electronic media.* (HSC 1998/242, p.4)

The pledge came formally into effect in April 1999.

In other areas of care, such as serious heart disease, there is evidence that delay costs lives. An editorial in *Heart* (1999; 81(6): 564) suggested the more than 500 patients may be dying each year while waiting to be admitted. So far the Government has not imposed stringent admission targets for this condition, although there were signs, when the editorial was published, that it might do so.

Finally, as we noted last year, it had been acknowledged that progress towards removing mixed-sex wards would be slow. In March 1999, a capital investment programme of over £1.1

billion was announced, including £40 million 'towards ending mixed-sex accommodation'. Clearly this still remains some way off.

Responsive services

We noted in last year's Review the establishment of the first three NHS Direct pilots in February 1998. The Government announced a year later that 'due to the phenomenal success story of NHS Direct' the scheme would be extended to cover 60 per cent of the country by the end of 1999, by adding new sites in south Yorkshire and south Humber, south west London, Bedfordshire and Hertfordshire, parts of Kent and Surrey and adding to the existing sites in Lancashire, Birmingham, Nottinghamshire, the West Country and Essex. Altogether, some £54 million was committed to NHS Direct in the financial year 1999/2000.

This second announcement added that:

> *Arrangements are now being made to set performance standards for NHS Direct call centres drawing on careful evaluation of experience so far and on best practice in other sectors. The Government is also planning on how to use the capacity of a national network to further improve the responsiveness of this service.* (PN 1999/0064, p.2)

In *NHS Direct – Final stage of national roll-out* (HSC 1999/028, 9 February 1999), the Executive set out the main features of a national service:

- *a national distinctive phone number (0845-46-47);*
- *a national performance management framework;*
- *national standards for service responsiveness, risk management and service quality;*
- *nationally procured decision support system(s) using nationally agreed clinical guidelines;*
- *a national staff competency framework;*
- *a national cost framework;*
- *national networking of providers and call management arrangements.* (HSC 1999/028, p.4)

However, the Circular does not indicate what the intended path of transition is from local pilots to the national design and, in particular, how the experience of the first- and second-wave projects – which employ a range of different approaches – will be used to develop a national system.

In part the Government's belief in the success of NHS Direct stemmed from the interim results of the monitoring carried out by the University of Sheffield. The Government used these results to justify the rapid expansion of the service, drawing on both the high satisfaction ratings and the diversion of some uses away from hospitals and towards self-care. The 'satisfaction' results are given in Table 1.4.

In February 1999, in *NHS Direct – Final stage of national roll-out* (HSC 1999/028), the Government indicated that there would be a third wave becoming operational by December 1999 and a final wave to become operational in summer/autumn 2000.

The high levels of satisfaction with the service would in themselves argue for its extension. However, a quite separate, but equally important measure of success, is whether or not the service had modified overall demands on the NHS. As Table 1.8 shows, it appears to have done so in nearly half the cases. As the first column indicates, nearly 40 per cent of those who might have gone to an A&E department did not do so, but a sizeable proportion was directed to the A&E department who would not have gone their of their accord. Altogether about half of those in the sample survey changed what they said they would do.

The Sheffield study does not reveal what the clinical or the cost implications of these changes were, so, at this stage, the overall impact of the service is far from clear. Furthermore, the use levels at all the sites were modest when the survey work was done.

TABLE 1.4

INTERIM RESULTS OF NHS DIRECT MONITORING

Percentage strongly agreeing or agreeing with the following statements (positive statements are in bold)

Aspect	*NHS Direct*
It was difficult to get through on the telephone	4
I was given exactly the right amount of advice needed**	**92**
I understood all the advice I was given	**98**
The advice I was given worked well in practice**	**90**
I was unhappy with the telephone advice I received**	9
I am satisfied with the explanation I was given**	**93**
I was given clear advice about when to get more help**	**95**
I was generally satisfied with the service**	**97**
I was made to feel I was wasting everyone's time*	7
I was not completely happy with the call**	6
The service I received could not be improved*	**64**

Notes

* $p<0.05$

** $p<0.005$

Source: Munro J *et al. Evaluation of NHS Direct first-wave sites: first interim report for the Department of Health*. Sheffield: University of Sheffield, December 1998, p.42.

The public health White Paper *Saving Lives: Our Healthier Nation* announced an extension to the service, NHS Direct Online, which will provide an interactive self-care guide and accredited information about hundreds of diseases and self-care groups. The first 100–200 public access points for both NHS Direct and NHS Direct Online are to be in place by April 2000. In addition, the experience of the telephone line will be used to develop an NHS Direct health care guide.

In April 1999 the Prime Minister announced a second initiative designed to make services more responses to users: the establishment of so-called 'walk-in' clinics. *NHS primary care walk-in centre* (HSC 1999/116), issued in May, indicated that up to £30 million would be available in the financial year 1999/2000 to support the development of around 20 sites with IT links with local practices. The key features of the centres are set out in Box 1.9.

BOX 1.9: KEY FEATURES OF WALK-IN CENTRES

- quick and convenient treatment as part of the modernised NHS
- high-quality care throughout the NHS, which is consistent and aimed at reducing variations
- positive experience for patients
- better health as well as health care – a healthier society
- partnership between NHS and each individual in achieving better health – promoting more autonomy.

Source: *NHS primary care walk-in centre* (HSC 1999/116), p.2.

In July it was announced that almost 100 bids had been received to be one of the first 20 pilots.

TABLE 1.5

COMPARISON OF EXPECTATION WITH ADVICE GIVEN

	Expectation A&E department	GP immediately	GP in next few days	Self-care only
A&E department	**57%**	13%	10%	14%
GP immediately	12%	**50%**	20%	13%
GP in next few days	11%	28%	**57%**	21%
Self-care only	15%	8%	15%	**46%**
Total = 100%	131	120	112	**269**

Source: Munro J *et al. Evaluation of NHS Direct first-wave sites: first interim report for the Department of Health.* Sheffield: University of Sheffield, December 1998, p.34.

COMPLAINTS

The second year of monitoring of the complaints procedures (*Handling Complaints: monitoring the NHS complaints procedure, England 1997/98*. London: Department of Health, 1999) found that the overall number of complaints had fallen relative to the previous year, although complaints had risen with respect to Family Health Services. In contrast, the Health Service Commissioner reported his workload to be rising – except in Wales – as Table 1.6 shows:

The NHS performance tables for 1997/98 include measures relating to the number of complaints and how they are handled. A significant proportion of trusts are recorded as not resolving complaints within the target time of four weeks. The vast majority of complaints, however, are resolved at this stage and do not go on to independent review.

We noted last year the Committee's irritation with so-called 'recidivist' trusts, which were found to persistently ignore the Ombudsman's findings. In its 1998 report the Committee concluded that the Government should provide details of specific actions taken in response to its recommendations. The Government response to the Committee's 1998 report (printed in an annex to the report) contains such a list. In respect of complaints, the Committee had identified the role of convenors as critical and had recommended further training. In its response the Government stated:

> *The Government recognises the importance of the role played by convenors (and others such as lay chairs) in the complaints process and the need for good quality training to enable them to carry out their role as effectively as possible. As the Committee notes, the Government has accepted that the Department has a continuing role to play in this area and the NHS Executive is currently considering, in conjunction with the Regional Offices, how to take this forward. A good practice guide for convenors is being developed which will be circulated to the NHS later this year. One of the key source documents for the guide is the Health Service Commissioner's memorandum which was put to the Committee as part of his evidence to them.*
> (Government response to the second report from the select committee on public administration (session 1997–98) on the report of the Health Service Ombudsman for 1996–97. London: The Stationery Office, 1998, p.ix)

TABLE 1.6

COMPLAINTS RECEIVED 1998/99 COMPARED WITH 1997/98 (BY REGION)

Region	*Complaints per 100,000 of population*	
	1998/99	*1997/98*
North Thames	6.92	7.18
South Thames	6.6	6.22
North West	5.3	4.22
South and West	4.47	4.25
West Midlands	4.36	4.06
Trent	4.02	3.73
Northern and Yorkshire	4.15	3.63
Anglia and Oxford	4.03	3.49
Totals for England	**5.11**	**4.71**
Scotland	4.24	3.83
Wales	4.83	5.1
Overall Totals	**5.02**	**4.65**

Source: Health Service Commissioner Annual Report for 1997/98. London: The Stationery Office, 1999.

The Government also indicated that it would follow-up the extensive regional variations in complaints reported last year and commission an independent evaluation of the complaints procedure as a whole. In November 1998 an evaluation project was announced. No findings were available at the time of going to press.

Compensation

We noted last year the massive rise in claims arising from alleged medical negligence. In April 1999 the Medical Protection Society – which represents about 45 per cent of GPs – reported that whereas there were 38 claims against GPs in 1989, by 1998 the number was 500. Furthermore, there was a 33-fold increase in the number of failed legal actions.

The NHS 1997/98 accounts confirmed the massive liability hanging over NHS trusts (totalling over £1.1 billion). In April 1999, as part of wide reforms of the legal system, new procedures were introduced to make it simpler, quicker and less expensive to pursue claims. The new fast track procedure for claims up to £15,000 limit the length of trial to one day, one expert per party and a maximum of 30 weeks to the trial date. A multi-track procedure is available for more complex cases. These reforms should cut litigation, if not compensation, costs to the NHS as well as to those making claims, but it is too early to judge their effect.

User surveys

The first ever national survey of NHS patients' views began in October 1998 and the results started to become available in April 1999. In commenting on them, the Government emphasised the fact that nine out of ten patients said they were happy with their GP's diagnosis. As Table 1.7 shows, the survey found even higher satisfaction levels with nurses.

However, in some areas, the survey found a substantial proportion of users who did not like what was on offer. Nearly half thought that they should have been referred earlier to a specialist and, among the younger age groups, sizeable minorities thought that the specialists did not have the necessary information when they were referred.

OVERALL

The emphasis on 'serving the consumer' has clearly changed since the new Government came to power, from attempts to make existing services become more responsive to introducing new ones. Furthermore, the Government is attempting to shift away from 'consumerism' towards a new relationship between service and user, one identified many years ago by Julian Tudor Hart – the patient as producer of health (Two paths for medical practice. *Lancet* 1992; 340 (8822): 772–75). The notion of the expert patient put forward in *Saving Lives: Our Healthier Nation* and the proposals for the extension of NHS Direct explicitly acknowledge the fact that many with chronic conditions come to know more about their conditions than their professional advisers, and that users in general are both keen and able to take some responsibility for their own health care needs. This perception was reinforced by the announcement in June 1999 of a series of research projects under the general title of 'Health in Partnership', involving:

- shared decision-making
- patient and public involvement in decisions about service development
- education and training implications of partnership between patients and professionals.

TABLE 1.7

WHETHER NURSE TREATED PATIENT WITH COURTESY AND RESPECT

		Sex	
	Total %	*Male %*	*Female %*
Courtesy and respect?			
Yes	99	99	99
No	1	1	1

Base: all seeing nurse in last 12 months

Source: National survey of NHS patients: General Practice 1998. London: Department of Health, 1999.

TABLE 1.8

WHETHER REFERRAL WAS SOON ENOUGH

		Sex	
	Total %	*Male %*	*Female %*
Seen as soon as necessary	56	53	58
Should have been seen a bit sooner	30	31	30
Should have been seen a lot sooner	14	16	12

Source: National survey of NHS patients: General Practice 1998. London: Department of Health, 1999.

TABLE 1.9

WHETHER SPECIALIST HAD NECESSARY INFORMATION

	Age (Female)				
	Under 25	*25–34*	*35–44*	*45–64*	*65+*
	%	%	%	%	%
Yes	66	74	77	83	89
No	23	15	14	9	5
Have not seen specialist yet	11	11	9	8	6

Source: National survey of NHS patients: General Practice 1998. London: Department of Health, 1999.

While that change is welcome, there are risks as well. The 'redirection' of patients reported for the first three NHS Direct pilots may lead to lower levels of service use and use of cheaper services, but it may (though the early figures do not suggest this) have the opposite effect if greater access to advice encourages more advice-seeking. Similarly, the availability of convenient services such as walk-in centres may add to the numbers seeking help for minor matters rather than diverting people from existing GP services. No-one knows what the balance will be, and there are no signs as yet that the Government is seeking to find out.

1.5 Clinical knowledge

Progress towards the improvement of clinical performance, through innovation and changes to existing structures, has been varied.

The New NHS set in motion a series of measures bearing on clinical performance, including new institutions (the National Institute for Clinical Excellence and the Commission for Health Improvement); new processes (national service frameworks, clinical governance and clinical performance measures); and changes to existing processes (self-regulation and lifelong learning for professionals). During this year, there have been varying degrees of progress towards bringing these changes into effect.

NEW INSTITUTIONS

As noted in Section 1.1, the creation of the Commission for Health Improvement requires legislation, so the implementation stage has not yet been reached. The Health Act provides for the Commission's establishment and contains a number of features that have a bearing on how it might work:

> *(a) the function of providing advice or information with respect to arrangements by Primary Care Trusts or NHS trusts for the purpose of monitoring and improving the quality of health care for which they have responsibility,*
> *(b) the function of conducting reviews of, and making reports on, arrangements by Primary Care Trusts or NHS trusts for the purpose of monitoring and improving the quality of health care for which they have responsibility,*
> *(c) the function of carrying out investigations into, and making reports on, the management, provision or quality of health care for which Health Authorities, Primary Care Trusts or NHS Trusts have responsibility,*
> *(d) the function of conducting reviews of, and making reports on, the management, provision or quality of, or access to or availability of, particular types of health care for which NHS bodies or service providers have responsibility, and*
> *(e) such functions as may be prescribed relating to the management, provision or quality of, or access to or availability of, health care for which prescribed NHS bodies or prescribed service providers have responsibility.* (s.20(1))

In particular, the Act gives the Secretary of State the power to specify the subjects of the Commission's inquiries; thus, the Government indicated in its statement on cancer that the Commission, when established, would be reviewing cancer care.

The Act does not, however, clarify the chief unknown about the Commission – how it will relate to the other agencies. As Angela Coulter points out elsewhere in this volume, the functions that the Commission seems likely to take on are similar to those of a number of other bodies. The Act neither specifies how these relationships should work, nor how the Commission will actually work to improve clinical standards. By the time this Review was written, no consultation document had appeared or ministerial speech been made to make the Government's intentions clearer.

Progress towards the establishment of the National Institute for Clinical Excellence has been somewhat faster. In January 1999, the NHS Executive issued a discussion document, *Faster Access to Modern Treatment: how NICE appraisal will work*. As the title itself implies, the emphasis at its launch was on the rapid spread of 'good value new treatments' across the country as a whole.

The discussion paper states that:

> 8. *The fundamental objective is to improve standards of patient care, and to reduce inequities in access to innovative treatment, by establishing a process which will*
> *i identify those new treatments and products which are likely to have a significant impact on the NHS, or which for other reasons would benefit from the issue of national guidance at an early stage*
> *ii enable evidence of clinical and cost effectiveness to be brought together to inform a judgement on the value of the treatment relative to alternative uses of resources in the NHS*
> *iii result in the issue of guidance on whether the treatment can be recommended for routine use in the NHS (and if so under what conditions or for which groups of patients) together with a summary of the evidence on which the recommendation is based*
> *iv avoid any significant delays to those sponsoring the innovation either in meeting any national or international regulatory requirements or in bringing the innovation to market in the UK.* (London: NHS Executive, 1999, p.2)

The paper sets out a process for new as well as existing interventions. In practice this proposed procedure might be hard to implement rigorously because the required information may not be available within the proposed timetable. Furthermore, the consultation paper does not appear to recognise that its decisions cannot be entirely technical in nature. Had it been in existence when Viagra was licensed, the Institute would have had to make recommendations on the drug's use. But, as Steve Dewar argues below, that decision involved a series of what were essentially political value judgements – made in that instance by a politician. The discussion paper does not define how political judgement will be brought to bear, or how the public will be involved in NICE decision-making. By the time of writing, the results of the consultation had not been published.

NATIONAL SERVICE FRAMEWORKS

As noted last year, mental health and coronary heart disease were selected as the first two services to be included in the national service frameworks programme. In December 1998 older people became the third subject and in April 1999 diabetes was added as the fourth.

The first published results of this new process appeared in November 1998 in *National Service Framework: Coronary Heart Disease: emerging findings*, which set out the scope of the programme in terms of the conditions it is intended to cover and the range of topics to be included. This report sets out a series of broad standards or areas for standards, examples of performance measures and a series of areas for further work.

By the time this Review went to press, no further results were available. However, in December 1998, *Cleft Lip and/or Palate Services* (HSC 1998/238) followed up an earlier report by the Clinical Standards Advisory Group, which had made a series of substantial recommendations as to how these services should be provided – a national service framework in all but name.

CLINICAL GOVERNANCE

Clinical Governance in the New NHS (HSC 1999/065) was issued in March 1999 and required, as a minimum, NHS trusts, health authorities and PCGs to:

> *By April 1999, identify lead clinicians for clinical governance and set up appropriate structures (including, for NHS Trusts, Board sub-committees) for overseeing clinical governance within their organisation;*
>
> *Agree with the relevant NHS Executive Regional Office (for NHS Trusts and Health Authorities) or Health Authorities (for PCGs and in due course PCTs) a process and timescale for conducting a baseline assessment of capability and capacity for implementing clinical*

governance;

Formulate an action plan in the light of this assessment;

Report on clinical governance arrangements within their Annual Reports for the year 1999/2000. (HSC 1999/065, p.4)

The Circular sees clinical governance as an integrating device at the local level:

20. Once it is recognised that this local organisational or service focus is central to developing clinical governance then it will be clear that many other initiatives and mechanisms must be connected so that the local drive to develop clinical governance is empowered and supported. (HSC 1999/065, p.8)

It also recognises that it is not just about processes:

Above all clinical governance is about changing organisational culture in a systematic and demonstrable way, moving away from a culture of 'blame' to one of learning so that quality infuses all aspects of the organisation's work. (HSC 1999/065, p.7)

A report, *Clinical governance in primary care: policy into practice* (NHS Confederation, 1999) confirmed the importance of this, concluding, on the basis of a national series of workshops, that:

Success requires commitment to:

- *meeting the needs of individual patients*
- *improving the public's health*
- *clinical quality*
- *clinical accountability*
- *multidisciplinary learning and development*
- *open and reflective practice*
- *respect and support colleagues*
- *an inclusive approach to working in partnership.* (p.1)

These may seem very demanding requirements, but a King's Fund study of the implementation of change in clinical practice by Michael Dunning and colleagues (*Experience, Evidence and Everyday Practice*. London: King's Fund, 1999) reinforces these findings. Its central conclusion was that change was possible and worthwhile, but it takes longer than expected and is expensive in terms of the commitment it requires. Furthermore, the process itself is complex and not reducible to a simple formula for success.

Progress therefore is likely to be slow. A survey by John Hayward and colleagues at the King's Fund of those leading clinical governance in London primary care groups found that while most had begun work, mainly in clinical areas, and that some thought it had great potential, all were concerned about the lack of resources – time and money – to do the job and also about their relationships with colleagues (Thin on the ground. *Health Service Journal* 26 August 1999: 26–27).

MEASURES OF CLINICAL PERFORMANCE

The Health Act 1999 provides for the introduction of the duty of quality, as foreshadowed in *The New NHS*, making chief executives of NHS trusts responsible for 'arrangements for the purpose of monitoring and improving the quality of health care [provided] to individuals'.

In June 1999, the first set of clinical performance indicators was published for England in *Quality and Performance in the NHS: clinical indicators* (London: Department of Health, 1999). The coverage is shown in Table 1.10.

TABLE 1.10

CLINICAL INDICATORS

Rates of death in hospital within 30 days of surgery by method of admission
Rates of death in hospital within 30 days of emergency admission with a hip fracture (neck of femur), for patients aged 65 and over
Rates of death in hospital within 30 days of emergency admission with a heart attack (myocardial infarction), for patients aged 50 and over
Rates of emergency readmission to hospital within 28 days of discharge from hospital
Rates of discharge to usual place of residence within 56 days of emergency admission from there with a stroke, for patients aged 50 and over
Rates of discharge to usual place of residence within 28 days of emergency admission from there with a hip fracture (neck of femur), for patients aged 65 and over

Source: *Quality and Performance in the NHS: clinical indicators.* London: Department of Health, 1999.

The values of the indicators produced showed very wide variations between trusts. In announcing the indicators, the Secretary of State was at pains to point out that they were not league tables; nor were they to be used by patients to shop around and travel for better treatment. Instead they were 'intended to help provide top quality treatment everywhere' (PR 1999/0355, 16 June 1999). But the link between indicator and 'top quality' is far from obvious.

Unlike their Scottish equivalents, the indicators are not accompanied by a statistical health warning, although in the Foreword to *Quality and Performance*, Sir Alan Langlands warns:

> *The indicators measure aspects of clinical care that impact on quality. Many factors, some of which are outside the direct control of hospitals, such as social circumstances and care by GPs, have an important bearing on the clinical results achieved by a particular hospital. These indicators do not therefore provide absolute measures on the outcomes of care but they identify where further investigation at a local level may be appropriate.*

He goes on to point out that:

> *Routinely available data on hospital activity, from which these indicators are derived, are not perfect. This is recognised and the data are being improved as new systems develop. The indicators here make the best possible use of existing information. They are a starting point and further work will support the development of the new Performance Assessment Framework and the National Service Frameworks.*

But what the end point will be remains unclear. While the range of indicators can be extended and their specification can undoubtedly be improved, some issues cannot be resolved in this way. The central issue is that, despite the Government's emphasis on the quality of care, what is meant by 'quality' remains undefined. By their nature the measures proposed can only capture some of the elements of the way that care is provided. Others may be captured by, for example, the NHS User Survey. This so far has been used to address broad questions rather than specific service issues, but this might change. We noted last year that consultations on the Patient's Charter found that professionals and users differed over the importance attached to different aspects of quality, the former naturally putting greater emphasis on clinical performance itself, and the latter more emphasis on choice and information.

When the views of users of cancer services are surveyed as part of the Government's cancer programme, they may well demonstrate diversity among users themselves as well as differences between professional and user views. This is not to say that either kind of measure should be rejected but, rather, that a lack of clarity remains as to how the information being provided through the new indicators should be used.

PROFESSIONAL REGULATION

The White Paper indicated the Government's intention to continue to rely on self-regulation. In the light of the Bristol case, however (see Klein R. Regulating the medical profession: doctors and the public interest. In: *Health Care UK 1997/98*), the medical profession acknowledges that changes have to be made. A paper from the Royal College of Physicians published in February 1999 acknowledged that:

> *Physicians have always aimed to maintain standards in their clinical practice and have generally achieved this. There is now a need not only to improve the methods for maintenance of standards but to demonstrate in an open fashion that individual physicians are indeed continuing in competent clinical practice.*
> (*Physicians maintaining good medical practice: Clinical governance and self-regulation.* London: Royal College of Physicians, 1999, p.1.)

It argued that a number of changes could be introduced immediately:

- *Annual, thorough two-way job plan review and appraisal of performance with a Clinical or Medical Director. The RCP will give advice on the job plan for all physicians.*
- *The introduction of regular continuing medical education of an interactive nature, based on a personal development plan, with assessment programmes being followed as they develop.*
- *Involvement in local or national audit of clinical outcome and process with evidence of action resulting if required.*
- *Introduction of a Royal College of Physicians Standards Adviser for each Trust or group of Trusts to assist in all of the above.*
- *Piloting of multidisciplinary peer assessment service reviews of clinical teams.* (p.1)

It also set out a much longer list of initiatives for further exploration. This paper and other similar announcements from professional bodies confirm that the professions have recognised the need for change.

The Government has also recognised this need: the Health Act gives the Government powers to reform the existing legislative framework and, in the light of a report from JM Consulting on the legislative structure of nursing regulation, it has already indicated that changes will be made. That report, published in August 1998, argued that despite reforms being made as recently as 1992 further changes were needed to address:

> - *weaknesses in the powers to protect the public from unsafe practice;*
> - *changes in the health care environment and in the education, structure and roles of the professions;*
> - *changed public expectations of the accountability of health professionals;*
> - *devolution within the United Kingdom.*
>
> (*The regulation of nurses, midwives and health visitors: report on a review of the Nurses, Midwives and Health Visitors Act 1997.* Bristol: JM Consulting, 1998)

It proposed a new Nurses and Midwives Act to streamline the regulatory structure and deal with these four issues. The Government has indicated that it will respond both to this report and an earlier one by the same consultants on Professions Allied to Medicine. However, Juan Baeza argues elsewhere in this volume that the Government's current plans do not go far enough: health care delivery is increasingly becoming a team, rather than an individual, responsibility both in hospital and community-based services, but the regulatory structure continues to ignore this.

RESEARCH AND DEVELOPMENT

As we noted in last year's Review, implementation of the Culyer proposals set in motion a process of reallocating finance for NHS R&D to parts of the NHS that had not received funds in the past. In November 1998 it was announced that £430 million was being allocated to R&D within the NHS, that the number of sites – hospitals and GP practices – where the money would be spent was being increased by 20 and that another 23 sites were to receive substantial increases to their funding. Thus there are some signs that the process of reallocation of resources away from the existing centres has begun. Typically, however, the amounts going to 'virgin' R&D organisations remain small, often less then £10,000.

The need for a re-orientation of R&D priorities emerges ever more strongly as the implications of the Government's agenda for the NHS become clearer. Throughout this Review we have pointed to gaps in knowledge and understanding – not of the specifics of health care delivery, on which the bulk of the R&D programme is spent, but of the process of implementing change and the design of whole systems of care as proposed in national service frameworks. These gaps are slowly being filled.

Saving Lives: Our Healthier Nation, for example, sets out the Government's intention to develop a research and development strategy for public health. A further significant development was the announcement of an R&D programme specifically focusing on the organisation of health care delivery. In contrast to existing programmes, which are focused largely on specific interventions, this will focus on 'service and organisation issues for all conditions, client groups and health care sectors'. Only limited information has so far emerged as to its scope and scale, but although in itself it will have little impact on the overall balance of the R&D programme, it represents a recognition that change is required.

DISSEMINATION

The development of a systematic process for disseminating clinical knowledge was one of the central features of the reforms introduced by the previous Government. Initially focused on support for purchasing decisions, it developed through the Cochrane centres and the cost-effectiveness bulletins into support for clinicians as well. In November the PRODIGY system was announced, which incorporates pharmaceutical advice and works online during the consultation process. This had been trialed extensively from 1995 onwards and is to be further developed to assist with chronic disease management.

The Government has this year announced two new processes to disseminate clinical knowledge – both of which have a bearing on the actual delivery of care. In February 1999 it was announced that the Chief Medical Officer was establishing a group to make recommendations on how the NHS can learn from experience when things go wrong, with the following terms of reference:

> *To examine the extent to which the National Health Service and its constituent organisations have the capability to learn from untoward incidents and service failures so that similar occurrences are avoided in the future. To draw conclusions and make recommendations.* (PR 1999/0065, 3 February 1999)

At the other end of the scale, a series of beacon awards were announced in September 1998 to celebrate success (*NHS Beacons*, HSC 1998/406). The beacon services initiative is intended to 'identify, celebrate and encourage learning from existing practice'. In its first year, the initiative is to focus on national priority areas including:

- waiting lists and times
- primary care
- mental health
- cancer services
- health improvement
- staff development.

About £10 million is to be used to:

- *make sure that each beacon service spends time spreading the word about its achievements, so that other services benefit;*
- *support other NHS Trusts and GP practices who want to start applying the lessons learned from visits to beacon sites;*
- *[ensure] the most successful beacon sites in each region will be selected to receive the special award of excellence the Nye Bevan award. They will be made each year.*

(HSC 1998/406, p.2)

In May 1999, well over 200 awards were announced, amounting to £50,000 for each trust and £4000 for each general practice. Also in May, 24 health improvement beacons were announced (each worth £20,000). These beacons are to enter into a learning agreement with the Department of Health, which encourages the spread of good practice by:

- *Participating in development networks and NHS events*
- *Participating in a programme of at least 6 'open days' each year*
- *Undertaking training for their own staff to further develop their skills in dissemination and training*
- *Acting as mentors of other similar services*
- *Participating in workshops, seminars and conferences*
- *Producing information on their service for the Learning Zone on NHSweb.*

(HSC 1999/0313, p.2)

Some of those selected as beacon service are to receive an Aneurin Bevan Award (or 'Nye'). There are to be eight regional prizes of £25,000 and a national prize of £50,000, to be spent on service development. The first awards were made in July 1999 to eight 'NHS trailblazers'.

INFORMATION STRATEGY

The NHS information and technology strategy, *Information for Health: an information strategy for the Modern NHS*, was published in September. In the same month HSC 1998/168 set out its main elements as follows:

- *lifelong Electronic Health Records for every person in the country*
- *round-the-clock online access to patient records and support on best clinical practice, for all NHS clinicians*
- *a National Electronic Library for Health to keep doctors and nurses, and other clinical professionals up to date with the latest clinical research and best practice at the time they need it*
- *integrated care for patients through GPs, hospitals and community services sharing information across the NHS information highway*
- *fast and convenient public access to information, advice and care through online information services and telemedicine*
- *more effective use of NHS resources by providing NHS planners and managers with the information they need.* (HSC 1998/168, p.3)

An initial £70 million was allocated from the Modernisation Fund to be spent in 1999/2000. To encourage take-up any expansion of local health information services funded in this way was excluded from the calculation of management costs. The hope is that the new information strategy for the NHS will help:

- *doctors, nurses and other clinicians to deliver better care by providing up-to-the-minute details of a patient's clinical history and current treatment, and access to the latest clinical research and best practice*
- *health service managers and planners to ensure the NHS spends its £40 billion budget in the most effective way and that all sectors of the NHS are working to the standards of the best*
- *patients to become more effectively involved in treatment decisions by providing accurate information about their clinical problems, and the public to stay fit and well by providing reliable health information.* (HSC 1998/168, p.6)

But whether these hopes will be fulfilled is another matter. During the year, the failure of large-scale IT systems at the Passport Office and the Department of Social Security made the headlines. As Justin Keen points out below, it is doubtful whether the NHS will do better. Indeed, there were already signs in mid-1999 that the target of having all GPs on the NHSnet will not be met.

PRIVATE SECTOR

The Health Act does not deal with the private health sector. A consultation document, *Regulating Private and Voluntary Health Care* (Department of Health, 1999), was published in June 1999. This proposed a new regulatory body to regulate the private and voluntary health sector, which would oversee the registration and inspection of private health care providers, deal with patients' complaints and publish inspection reports. It also proposed that private patients should have access to clinical and non-clinical information on areas such as staffing, facilities available and the range of services provided.

Although the consultation document recognises that changes are required to the current regulatory regime, it contains no description of the current role of the private sector. In particular, it ignores the fact that the NHS is itself a private care provider – or provider of facilities for private care – and also, particularly in mental health, makes extensive use of them.

In July 1999 the Health Committee published *The Regulation of Private and other Independent Healthcare* (London: The Stationery Office, 1999), which did tackle the broader picture as well as focusing on particular problem areas such as cosmetic surgery, children's services and mental health. It also recognised the need to address private work within the NHS by proposing that private facilities within an NHS trust should be required to function within the clinical procedures and management of that trust.

The Committee argued for an independent regulator for health care outside the NHS, but one with a wider role than that envisaged by the Government. Overall, these and other Committee recommendations are designed to offer similar standards of protection to private sector users as those enjoyed within the NHS or from other service providers, and also to introduce some explicit rules bearing on private sector/NHS relationships (such as the transmission of information between private and NHS GPs). By the time of writing, the Government response had not been published.

OVERALL

A year after our first overview of Labour's proposals, the process of implementation has moved on by a modest degree but nothing of substance has emerged. The tensions within the different approaches have yet to emerge strongly – in particular between the role of the centre and the locality. But, as Steve Dewar has emphasised (*Clinical Governance under Construction*. London: King's Fund, 1999), as the various organisations and processes referred to above start becoming effective, these tensions will grow. The more guidelines appearing from the centre, either through the work of NICE or the national service frameworks, the greater the task – in time and costs terms – both of implementing them and monitoring how the implementation is proceeding. The King's Fund work referred to above emphasises the importance of 'local' ownership when change in clinical delivery systems is being made. As the NICE paper recognises, some interventions require substantial organisational and clinical change if they are to be properly introduced. These not only require the personal commitment that the work cited above pinpointed as a key requirement, but also financial and organisational commitment, which will inevitably pose issues of priority.

Choices will have to be made locally as to where effort should be focused. But such a pragmatic approach will tend to conflict with the Government's aim of introducing a greater degree of consistency between different parts of the NHS. We return to this issue in Section 2.2.

Part 2 Commentary

2.1 Finance and efficiency

The Government has made additional finance available to the NHS, but cost pressures remain.

The financial framework for the NHS was largely set by the announcements made in 1998 following the Comprehensive Spending Review. The large cash injection announced in 1998 appeared to remove the immediate risk of financial strains appearing. Furthermore, in November 1998 the Chancellor announced an extra £250 million for the NHS on a one-off basis. These increases represented a substantially higher increase in real terms over the figures of the previous two years, the low level of which went some way towards explaining why we reported last year that many health authorities and trusts were in serious financial difficulty.

The NHS summarised accounts for England for the financial year 1997/98 showed that 86 out of the 100 health authorities had a deficit at the end of the year – slightly down on the previous year's total. Subsequent monitoring by the Executive suggested that the number of authorities with serious financial problems – estimated to be 29 at the end of 1997/98 – had dropped to 19 by the end of the third quarter of 1998/99. At the end of 1997/98 149 trusts were in deficit, of which 99 were considered to be material. Seven out of the nine trusts with deficits over £10 million were in London.

In November, health authority allocations were announced. Although all authorities enjoyed real terms increases, a substantial part of the overall increase in the NHS budget was reserved for the so-called Modernisation Fund (as John Appleby shows in Datawatch, p.152). During the year, a series of announcements were made linking particular service developments to the Fund; by far the largest amount was targeted on waiting lists, followed by the establishment of primary care groups and improvements to primary care.

SUPPLEMENTARY FINANCE

We noted last year both the Government's commitment to a tax-funded NHS and its readiness to use lottery monies to fund healthy living centres. Although these are not designed to provide mainstream health services, they will offer patients facilities that might also be funded from the NHS. In March 1999, the Government went further by announcing that £150 million from the New Opportunities Fund would be devoted to the improvement of cancer services. This will be used for scanners and x-ray machines, new treatments, better prevention and providing improved access to screening.

In November 1998, the Road Traffic (NHS Charges) Bill was published, which provided for:

- the transfer of responsibility for collecting charges from hospitals to the Secretary of State for Health
- a centralised, national administrative system to collect charges
- the introduction of a simple, national tariff of charges to mirror the real costs of treatment
- reviews and appeals against decisions
- powers to gather information needed to collect charges
- ensuring that the money collected is transferred to the hospital that provided the treatment and care.

The Act came into effect in April 1999; the Government claimed that it would provide £100 million a year extra income for the NHS.

In respect of charges, however, the Government decided to raise less than it might have. As from 1 April 1999, prescription charges were raised from £5.80 to £5.90, the lowest increase for 20 years, free sight tests were restored and the value of optical vouchers was increased by 18 per cent.

CAPITAL FINANCE

The Government continued to press ahead with more schemes under the private finance initiative. In November 1998 a total investment programme of £2.2 billion was announced and a further tranche in July 1999 brought the total committed to over £3 billion.

In May 1999, the National Audit Office published the first official appraisal of this method of hospital procurement: *The PFI Contract for the new Dartford and Gravesham Hospital* (The Stationery Office, 1999). This makes it clear that the hospital will cost more than the service it replaces and that the trust overestimated the savings it would make relative to the public sector alternative. The National Audit Office also found that less than one-fifth of the local GPs surveyed thought the new hospital would meet patients' needs 'fairly well' or satisfactorily. Nearly three out of five thought it would be unsatisfactory in this respect.

In July 1999, a Government-wide review of the private finance initiative was published. It announced a new organisation, Partnerships UK, which is to act as project manager for PFI deals – although only if invited. Also, although Partnerships UK will not act as a bank, it will offer a range of financial facilities to public sector bodies. The impact of this proposal on the NHS remains to be seen.

In May a capital strategy was announced. This was described as the 'first ever capital investment strategy for the NHS and social services', prepared in response to the requirement set out in the Treasury's *Stability and Investment for the Long Term: Economic and Fiscal Strategy Report 1998* (The Stationery Office, 1998) that each Department should produce an investment strategy. In fact, the document fell short of being that. Far from being a strategy, it is an incoherent re-statement of a series of commitments that the Government has entered into, such as the modernisation of A&E departments, without actually developing a strategy for emergency care as a whole. Similarly, the strategy document records the setting up of a national beds inquiry in September 1999 after the Government had already committed over £2 billion of capital investment in hospitals.

Some of this had already been committed to A&E facilities. In September 1998 it was announced that one in four departments would be modernised. In February 1999, it was stated that one in three A&E departments would receive support for modernisation of facilities. In March it was announced that all A&E departments would be modernised, and at the same time a team led by Mike Lambert (A&E consultant at Norfolk and Norwich) was established to spread good practice. In May details of spending on 149 departments were released, including:

> *the re-design and re-decoration of older, outdated departments as well as improvements in a wide range of innovative areas including:*
> *– new diagnostic and other equipment to ease assessment of patients;*
> *– more observation wards and admissions units to reduce waiting time in A&E;*
> *– greater use of telemedicine to link up community hospitals in rural areas with larger city centres hospitals to ensure wider access to expert medical opinion;*
> *– better facilities for children including separate waiting areas with playrooms, and separate assessment and treatment areas;*
> *– improved security measures to better protect staff and patients from violence and abuse.* (PR 1999/0325)

EFFICIENCY AND PERFORMANCE

As we noted last year, although the new Government has abandoned the main instruments used by its predecessor to extract efficiency gains from the NHS, the commitment to do so remains, albeit as one of several categories of performance measures. The revised NHS performance assessment framework was published in March 1999. As the Government indicated when the consultation document was published in 1998, this is intended to provide a more rounded account of the NHS's achievements than the previous emphasis on a single efficiency index and we look at it in the context of overall accountability in Section 2.3. The high level indicator set contains five efficiency indicators (see Table 2.1).

TABLE 2.1

EFFICIENCY INDICATORS 1999/2000

Day case rate
Length of stay in hospital (case-mix adjusted)
Unit cost of maternity (adjusted)
Unit cost of caring for patients in receipt of specialist mental health services (adjusted)
Generic prescribing

How these relate, if they relate at all, to the continuing target for efficiency gains is unclear. The Treasury consultation document on output and performance analyses suggests that they are to be sought by:

- reducing variation in NHS trust unit costs
- procurement savings
- reducing management costs
- trust asset sales.

In November 1998, the Executive published the first set of comparative costs information, the *1998 Reference Costs*, which sets out for all NHS trusts the costs per case for most elective treatments.

As the document itself helpfully points out, '... the NHS is not a manufacturer of widgets' and consequently costs are influenced by the nature of the patients themselves and the treatment they are offered. The adjustments to the data – which are presented in health resource groups – do not allow perfectly for either of these factors. The costs vary by very large, indeed unbelievable, amounts, suggesting that although in principle they have been drawn up in a similar way, in practice they have not been.

But even if the figures are accurate, it remains unclear how the differences will be exploited to extract savings. Alan Milburn's introduction to the document suggests that:

> *In combination with information on quality, unit costs will help NHS trusts to identify best practice, reduce costs and free resources for reinvestment.*

In themselves unit costs do not identify best practice and information on quality at the level of the individual procedure is not available. So while a start has been made, there is a very long way to go before the data can be effectively used for these purposes.

In June 1999, the results of a Cabinet Office review of NHS procurement were announced. This review recommended the establishment of an NHS Purchasing and Supply Agency from next April; that experienced NHS procurement staff should be used to provide a dedicated local source of advice; that all NHS trusts identify a lead director for procurement; and that all NHS trusts draw up procurement strategies with targets for delivering savings of at least 3 per cent a year.

Claims of improvements in NHS procurement efficiency represent a triumph of hope over experience, as a series of reports from the National Audit Office has demonstrated. The Cabinet Office report on which the changes are based notes that over the years a series of weaknesses has been persistently identified:

- *Fragmented purchasing – a need for more joint contracting.*
- *Lack of common specifications – a reluctance to agree standards of regular use items, a precursor to joint contracting.*
- *Incomplete management information – a lack of reliable data on usage, lines purchased, supplier performance and price levels.*
- *Insufficient management attention – procurement tended to be of peripheral interest to senior management.*
- *Inadequate storage facilities – stores were small, disparate and poorly controlled.*
- *A need for specialist well trained supplies managers.*

Even if the changes are effective, improvements will prove slow to realise against this background.

MANAGEMENT COSTS

In *NHS Trust Management Trusts: target setting and definitions for NHS Trusts* (HSC 1999/040, 19 February 1999), the Government continued to demonstrate its commitment 'to increasing the proportion of every pound spent in the NHS on patient care'. The Circular suggests that 'the abolition of the internal market, and further benchmarking, should enable, over five years from 1997/98, £1 billion which would otherwise have been spent on management and administration to be spent on patient care. To date, reductions in 1997/98 and 1998/99 mean that ... an estimated £240 million has been redirected from management towards patient care'. It then goes on to affirm that NHS trusts would be required to reduce their management costs by £100 million over the next three years (para.4). The further savings are to be achieved by targeting trusts with proportionately higher management costs and seeking savings from trusts undergoing mergers. As John McClenahan notes below, the latter expectation may be disappointed. However, the Circular goes on to suggest that more savings can be made by sharing services and pooling functions between trusts – although without specifying how much might be gained in this way.

A similar Circular was directed at health authorities and primary care groups. This stated, however, that there would be no targets for further net reduction in health authority costs over the next three years.

PHARMACEUTICAL COSTS

As noted last year, the existing Pharmaceutical Price Regulation Scheme had to be renegotiated. In July 1999, a new five-year agreement was announced, which, it was claimed, would save some £200 million a year or about 4.5 per cent of current expenditure on drugs. In addition to this voluntary agreement, the Government took powers within the Health Act 1999 to control the price of medicines. The Act provides for the Secretary of State to either limit prices or profits and to impose fines if any regulations made under these powers are contravened.

The total bill is of course also heavily influenced by prescribing patterns. The creation of primary care groups and the capping of prescribing costs overall mean that the financial constraint is now a tougher one. In addition, as noted in Section 1.5, the PRODIGY system has been introduced to support effective prescribing.

FRAUD

In December 1998, the Government published *Countering Fraud, the NHS Counter Fraud Strategy* (HSC 1998/0576). The aims are to:

- *reduce fraud to an absolute minimum within 10 years,*
- *hold it permanently at that level and thereby*
- *free up resources for better patient care.* (p.3)

The Government's determination to reduce fraud was further demonstrated in the form of a campaign, announced in March 1999, aimed at reducing prescription fraud by patients by 50 per cent by the end of 2002/03, as well as contractor fraud by a substantial amount. In April 1999 the Minister of State for Health, John Denham announced that every health authority and trust will have a professional counter fraud specialist to investigate the local incidence of fraud. These specialists, along with regional and national staff, will form the Counter Fraud Operational Service.

PAY AND HUMAN RESOURCES

Claims for substantial increases in pay are potentially the largest drain on the extra resources the Government has made available to the NHS. We noted last year the signs that the NHS was finding it hard to recruit and retain professional staff, particularly nurses, and that it accepted the case presented to it by the Standing Advisory Committee on the Medical Workforce that the number of doctors should be increased. In September 1998 Alan Milburn announced a £50 million recruitment plan involving:

- *Extra training places for nurses, including new funding to expand the number of part-time pre-registration nursing and midwifery courses.*
- *Targeting nurses who have left the profession. Extra cash paid in bursaries will enable 2700 Enrolled Nurses to retrain and return to the NHS with full qualifications over the next three years.*
- *Broadening the career structure for nurses. Over 1000 existing NHS staff such as healthcare assistants will be able to become qualified nurses – with all of their income protected during training – thanks to extra cash over the next three years.*
- *Improving nurses' working conditions. By April 2000 every local employer must have systems to monitor accidents and violence against staff, and have plans to cut these incidents. There will also be a centrally supported drive to ensure that the NHS becomes a family friendly employer of nurses.* (PR 1998/396)

In January a £5 million campaign 'Nurses Make a Difference' was launched, with nationwide advertising and the establishment of a 24-hour nursing line. Less than a month later, the Secretary of State was announcing 'an excellent response'. Furthermore the Department of Health had carried out a survey among nurses not currently working in the NHS, which suggested that one in five were planning to return and another three out of five might be persuaded to do so if conditions of work could be made more flexible.

These essentially short-term measures were accompanied by measures announced in *Widening Access to Nursing and Midwifery Education and Training* (HSC 1998/182, 16 October 1998) to broaden access to nursing and midwifery education and training, which included non-means tested bursaries for enrolled nurses, new secondment opportunities, and the expansion of part-time and more flexible diploma programmes.

As for doctors, the 1998 Medical Practice Committee survey suggested no major change in recruitment patterns to general practice. The Government was able to announce a 7.7 per cent increase in the number of GP registrars, but this only put the numbers back to the 1993 level. Thus, unless the increase is sustained, it will be hard to maintain the present labour force.

In attempting to form its view of the recruitment situation, the Pay Review Body for Doctors and Dentists found that there was the familiar sharp difference of opinion between the Health Departments on the one hand and the BMA on the other. While the Departments cited the Medical Practices Committee survey findings, the BMA put more emphasis on long-term factors, including the increase in the workload (an 18.4 per cent increase in consultations over ten years), the long-term decline in GMP registrars and the fall in certificates issued by the Joint Committee for Postgraduate Training in General Practice. Overall, the Review Body concluded there was no recruitment crisis but indicated it intended to keep the situation under review.

There is no dispute that recruitment and retention must be taken into account. However there always has been disagreement about what other factors are relevant. The tension lies between the (employers') view that these are all that matter and the (employees') view that comparability with other professions is relevant.

As the Review Body records, the Prime Minister wrote to it in July to propose certain changes in the way its recommendations would be handled. The letter attempted to redefine the framework within which the Review Body works, suggesting that:

> *... within the new CSR approach, the key considerations would be recruitment, retention and motivation of our remit groups; the Department's output targets for the delivery of services; the Department's three year expenditure limits; and the Government's inflation target. While departments might still ask us to address other specific considerations in the evidence they put to us, the ones he had identified set the strategic framework that Departments would have to work with and that we would therefore need to recognise in considering our recommendations ...* (Review Body on Doctors' and Dentists' Remuneration 28th Report, para.1.16)

Subsequently the Minister for Health wrote suggesting new terms of reference. The Review Body, however, argued that it should continue to be independent and to weight all the evidence it received equally. In particular:

> *... we would continue to be free, after careful consideration of all the evidence, to ... [recommend] ... awards that we felt were appropriate, and that there was no suggestion that we should feel constrained to limit our recommendations.* (Review Body on Doctors' and Dentists' Remuneration 28th Report, para.1.17)

The new terms of reference – which also apply to the Review Body for Nurses – reflect a compromise between these positions, and are detailed in Box 2.1. The public spending and macro-economic elements are set out only too clearly, but the need to consider motivation, as well as recruitment and retention, is also included. Both Bodies refer in their reports to their determination to make 'fair' recommendations.

In February, the NHS Executive set out proposals for modernising the NHS pay system in *Agenda for Change* (HSC 1999/035). The paper states:

> *The NHS pay system needs to change. It needs to reflect the world of 1999 rather than the world of 1948. It needs to reward the actual responsibilities that staff take on rather than the job title they work under. It needs to offer the prospect of higher, inclusive, salaries rather than relying on expensive, outdated, inflexible special allowances. It needs to provide flexibility so jobs can be designed to suit patient needs rather than with rigid demarcation lines on what staff think they are allowed to do.* (HSC 1999/035, p.3)

It sets out only in the most general terms how these requirements should be met. It goes on, however, to define three aims:

- *enables staff to give their best for patients, working in new ways and breaking down traditional barriers*
- *pays fairly and equitably for work done, with career progression based on responsibility, competence and satisfactory performance*
- *simplifies and modernises conditions of service, with national core conditions and considerable local flexibility.* (HSC 1999/035, p.6)

and then sets out three proposals:

- *core conditions of service for all staff, with a single national negotiating council – the General Whitley Council*
- *A national job evaluation framework*
- *Clear and simplified arrangements for pay spines.* (HSC 1999/035, pp.10–11)

BOX 2.1: DOCTORS AND DENTISTS REVIEW BODY REVISED TERMS OF REFERENCE

The Review Body on Doctors' and Dentists' Remuneration is independent. Its role is to make recommendations to the Prime Minister, the Secretary of State for Health, the Secretary of State for Scotland and the Secretary of State for Wales on the remuneration of doctors and dentists taking any part in the National Health Service.

In reaching its recommendations, the Review Body is to have regard to the following considerations:

– the need to recruit, retain and motivate doctors and dentists;
– the Health Departments' output targets for the delivery of services, as set out by the Government;
– the funds available to the Health Departments as set out in the Government's Departmental Expenditure Limits;
– the Government's inflation target.

The Review Body may also be asked to consider other specific issues.

The Review Body is also required to take careful accounts of the economic and other evidence submitted by the Government, staff and professional representatives and others.

Reports and recommendations should be submitted jointly to the Secretary of State for Health, the Secretary of State for Scotland, the Secretary of State for Wales and the Prime Minister. (p.ii)

Source: Review Body on Doctors' and Dentists' Remuneration 28th Report. London: Stationery Office, 1999.

It then argues that there should be more scope to move away from national grades and boundaries and to set pay bands within national guidance, including scope for pay to adjust to the local labour market. In this and other ways, the paper seeks to extend local freedoms to determine conditions of employment – in other words moving in the same direction as local pay. Not surprisingly, therefore, the negotiations to achieve these ends proved slow and no progress had been announced by the time this Review went to press.

The House of Commons Health Select Committee published *Future NHS Staffing Requirements*, a wide-ranging if short inquiry making a series of proposals for improving workforce planning as well as pay. Like the Pay Review Body it concluded that the link between the Government's service plans and staff requirements was unclear. It therefore recommended:

> *... a major review of current planning procedures which should pay particular regard to their rationalisation and eventual replacement by an integrated planning system. We think it necessary that any new system should not only incorporate the national overview currently provided by the sub-group of the NHSE, but also actively promote a national strategy for workforce planning which, allowing for local conditions, brings a sense of consistency and cohesion at present notable for its absence (paragraph 36).* (p.xlii)

And:

> *... it is time now to reorganise the pay review body system in order to inculcate a greater sense of team spirit within the NHS. We therefore recommend its replacement with the*

establishment of a single body charged with the task of reviewing the pay of all NHS professionals. This body should have within its remit all NHS staff, for example, clinical scientists and ancillary workers, who are not included in the current pay review bodies. The independence of the body should be secure and unassailable (paragraph 158). (p.xliii)

The Government response, *Future Staffing Requirements* (Cm. 4379. London: Stationery Office, 1999), stated the Government's 'determination to make progress in this area' and in particular noted that a workforce planning branch for the whole of the NHS had just been set up. It accepts however that 'more fundamental improvements to workforce planning are required' and that a major review is to be launched 'in the near future'.

In May 1999 the Executive published *Modernising Health and Social Services: Developing the workforce*, which stated that the Government was committed to:

- *achieving greater coherence between strategies for service development and workforce planning*
- *improving workforce planning systems at all levels, across the whole range of services – in primary and secondary care, across agencies, and across professional and vocational boundaries.*

Although the document makes many proposals bearing on the latter, it fails to make the link between service and workforce planning – or between them and the capital strategy. There remains a long way to go before all elements of the provision of health care services are effectively planned for – individually and in relation to each other. But if the Government is serious in trying to link the pay bill to its 'output targets for the delivery of services', it is precisely such an integration that is required.

An indication of the difficulties appeared in March 1999 when it was announced that 350 doctors qualifying in obstetrics and gynaecology would fail to find a job after completing their specialist training. The numbers in training had been based on the assumption that consultant numbers would continue to rise rapidly, but the rapid growth experienced up to 1997 did not continue at the same rate. This might be regarded as a simple failure to make the proper links between service and workforce planning, but in fact it reveals a more fundamental weakness – that medical training is so long and rapidly becomes so specialised that no forecasting system can be relied upon.

CHANGING THE NHS SERVICE BUNDLE

Long-term care

As noted above, the majority report of the Royal Commission argued for a redefinition of the NHS boundary, which would bring personal care within the ambit of the NHS and, as a result, increase NHS spending. As noted in Section 1.2, the Government has yet to respond to this proposal.

Dentistry

Previous Reviews have noted the gradual disappearance of adult dentistry from the NHS menu and the Government's determination to counter this trend, using the framework of the Primary Care Act 1997 to establish a series of pilots designed to try out new ways of providing the service. This determination was further evidenced by a second wave of personal dental service pilots announced in January 1999. As John Hayward points out elsewhere in this volume, it remains to be seen how determined the Government is to make NHS dental care readily available to all those who wish to have it. A new dental strategy has been promised, which should shed some light on this.

Drugs

The licensing of Viagra in September 1998 appeared to take the Government by surprise. The Standing Medical Advisory Committee had already been asked for advice and interim guidance was issued in September. The Committee then offered further advice and a period of consultation began in January 1999.

When announcing the consultation, the Secretary of State said:

We issued interim guidance on Viagra in September, a day before it received a European licence. The guidance advised doctors not to prescribe Viagra until further notice. We took this position because of our concern that Viagra could become a serious drain on NHS funds, due to the huge amount of attention given to this drug. Since then, we have been gathering advice to develop today's policy proposals.

Impotence is in itself neither life threatening, nor does it cause physical pain. It can, in exceptional circumstances, cause psychological distress. Until the advent of Viagra, NHS expenditure on this condition has been limited because of the nature of the treatments available.

Now that the treatment is available in tablet form, the cost of treating impotence could escalate. The cost could increase tenfold or even more. To limit this impact, we propose controls which reflect the priority given to treatment for impotence, and reflect its current level of expenditure. (PR 1999/0037, 21 January 1999)

Following the consultation, the Secretary of State put out new guidelines in May, setting out the categories of men who could receive treatment:

Men treated for prostate cancer
Men suffering from spinal cord injury
Men treated for kidney failure
Men with diabetes
Men with Multiple Sclerosis
Men with single gene neurological disease
Men with spina bifida
Men who have had polio
Men with Parkinson's disease
Men with severe pelvic injury
For other men who are caused severe distress by impotence, it is proposed that treatment should be available in exceptional circumstances only after a specialist assessment in a hospital
(PR 1999/0315, p.1)

This list was longer than was originally proposed, reflecting points made in the consultation process. In the same month, the maker of Viagra, Pfizer, won a case in the High Court, which successfully challenged the Secretary of State's interim guidance, essentially on procedural grounds. It did not, however, lead to the final May advice being overturned. Consequently the restrictions surrounding the use of Viagra seem set to continue. As Steve Dewar points out below, the significance of the Secretary of State's decision goes far beyond this particular drug: it is the first time that any Government minister had endorsed a rationing decision in terms of the need to limit public expenditure.

OVERALL

The extra resources announced in the 1998 Comprehensive Spending Review meant that the NHS would enjoy a higher rate of growth than it had done in the previous two years. But, over and above the pressures described here from higher pay awards, the NHS is faced with cost pressures from the introduction of the national minimum wage and European Union working time directives, the costs of providing against the year 2000 bug in computer systems, and the familiar pressures arising from new drug developments.

2.2 Equity

The NHS has a long-standing commitment to 'equity', but 'equal access for equal need' may not be the right objective.

As we noted last year, and as has been confirmed this year, the Government has placed reduction in health inequalities near the top of its priorities. As Sir Donald Acheson argued in his report, these must be addressed by a very wide range of measures bearing on the economic, social and physical environment. His proposals for the NHS were limited, in part because the report recognises that health care is itself only one contributor to good health and in part because the allocation of resources within the NHS has, insofar as the process has been explicit, followed the equity principle of equal access for equal need. In large measure, therefore, Sir Donald's proposals were designed to ensure that access is in fact equal.

But, as his report acknowledges, it is not easy to determine whether access is equal or not. As this Section of the Review noted last year, although there is a great deal of evidence on variations in use, little of it allows for variations in need and other factors that might influence service take-up. Accordingly, of the 11 recommendations Sir Donald directed at the NHS, nearly all are concerned with processes and research rather than specific services or obstacles to access.

For despite the venerable nature of the principle of equal access for equal need, it continues to be hard to implement in practice. The obstacles are in part technical and we consider some of these below. But they also reflect more fundamental difficulties stemming from the overall way in which the NHS is now being run, and which pose issues of principle around the extent to which equality in respect of service and use should in fact be a target at all. We begin, however, with financial allocations, where practical problems continue to arise.

FINANCIAL ALLOCATIONS

For more than 20 years, there have been continuing efforts to equalise resources relative to need in different parts of England. Nevertheless, the technical task remains only partially solved. In November 1998, a wide-ranging review of the formula used for making cash allocations to health authorities and primary care groups was announced. It will be carried out alongside a similar review of the formulae used to allocate finance to local authorities. In the meantime, some small adjustments were made to the existing formula:

- the specialty cost weights in the HCHS age adjustment were updated. A new need adjustment for prescribing was introduced, so that the allocation for drugs costs more accurately reflect the need in each health authority
- a monetary adjustment was introduced to supplement the formula for the extra costs of interpretation, advocacy and translation services.

In addition, the Government indicated, in line with another of Sir Donald's recommendations, that it wished to see health authorities reach their 'fair share' capitation targets as soon as possible. In line with that intention, the increase in allocations announced in November 1998 varied considerably (see Table 2.2). In 1999/2000, 97 per cent of authorities are within 5 per cent of their target.

TABLE 2.2

1999/2000 HEALTH AUTHORITY ALLOCATIONS (INCLUDING TARGETED FIGURE FOR HAZs)

Health authorities	*% increase*
Northern and Yorkshire	
Bradford	4.63
Calderdale and Kirklees	4.07
County Durham	4.48
East Riding	4.31
Gateshead and South Tyneside	4.34
Leeds	4.20
Newcastle and North Tyneside	4.31
North Cumbria	4.18
North Yorkshire	3.91
Northumberland	4.20
Sunderland	4.37
Tees	4.41
Wakefield	4.20
Trent	
Barnsley	5.22
Doncaster	4.43
Leicestershire	4.53
Lincolnshire	3.82
North Derbyshire	3.88
North Nottinghamshire	4.11
Nottingham	4.78
Rotherham	4.66
Sheffield	4.27
South Derbyshire	4.29
South Humber	2.90
Anglia and Oxford	
Bedfordshire	4.85
Berkshire	4.77
Buckinghamshire	4.54
Cambridge and Huntingdon	4.10
East Norfolk	3.81
North West Anglia	4.25
Northamptonshire	3.80
Oxfordshire	4.77
Suffolk	2.92
North Thames	
Barking and Havering	4.00
Barnet	3.98
Brent and Harrow	3.21
Camden and Islington	4.43
Ealing, Hammersmith and Hounslow	4.06
East and North Hertfordshire	3.99
East London and the City	5.48
Enfield and Haringey	4.12
Hillingdon	3.86
Kensington, Chelsea and Westminster	6.06
North Essex	3.97
Redbridge and Waltham Forest	2.89
South Essex	4.62
West Hertfordshire	3.79
South Thames	
Bexley and Greenwich	2.88
Bromley	3.89
Croydon	4.12
East Kent	3.77
East Surrey	2.92
East Sussex, Brighton and Hove	3.76
Kingston and Richmond	2.93
Lambeth, Southwark and Lewisham	4.50
Merton, Sutton and Wandsworth	3.76
West Kent	3.81
West Surrey	2.91
West Sussex	3.99
South and West	
Avon	4.09
Cornwall and Isles of Scilly	3.22
Dorset	2.91
Gloucestershire	2.90
Isle of Wight	3.38
North and East Devon	2.92
North and Mid Hampshire	3.80
Portsmouth and SE Hampshire	4.05
Somerset	3.81
South and West Devon	3.05
Southampton and SW Hampshire	3.98
Wiltshire	3.78

West Midlands	
Birmingham	3.90
Coventry	4.66
Dudley	4.06
Herefordshire	3.86
North Staffordshire	4.70
Sandwell	4.73
Shropshire	3.92
Solihull	4.22
South Staffordshire	3.81
Walsall	4.75
Warwickshire	2.92
Wolverhampton	4.54
Worcestershire	3.78
North West	
Bury and Rochdale	4.48
East Lancashire	3.97
Liverpool	4.26
Manchester	3.42
Morecambe Bay	2.89
North Cheshire	2.92
North West Lancashire	3.91
Salford and Trafford	4.12
Sefton	4.13
South Cheshire	3.82
South Lancashire	2.91
St Helen's and Knowsley	4.27
Stockport	4.08
West Pennine	4.19
Wigan and Bolton	4.56
Wirral	4.09
England	4.00

Source: PN 1998/0500.

The impact of the work on the allocation formula is not expected to be felt until after the end of the period covered by the Comprehensive Spending Review. However, according to *Reducing Inequalities*, the review of the formula has the fundamental objective of contributing a reduction in avoidable health inequalities and will include the impact of ethnicity on health and the cost of providing services.

In one area, however, the Government has committed itself to immediate change. We noted in last year's Review that research by Alan Maynard and Karen Bloor had revealed considerable disparities in the levels of financial resources available for general medical services. The Department of Health has committed itself to attempting to redress this imbalance by setting an explicit target. Its 'agreement' with the Treasury includes the following commitment:

> (v) *Improve access to and quality of primary care services through investment in line with locally agreed Primary Care Investment Plans. Key targets are:*
> *a) progress towards a national average annual increase of 1% whole-time-equivalent GPs by 2002, using a range of new initiatives and with local variations to take account of the need to concentrate on deprived and remote areas;*
> *b) increase investment in practice staff – 500 new practice nurses will be appointed by 2002;*
> *c) improve the quality of primary care premises, targeted towards areas of deprivation, resulting in improvements to 1,000 premises nationally by 2002.*
> (*Public services for the future: modernisation, reform, accountability: comprehensive spending review: public service agreements 1999–2002.* London: The Stationery Office, 1998.)

The Treasury paper, *The Government's Measures of Success: output and performance analyses*, fails to provide a measure of what would constitute a more equitable distribution – it refers only to total numbers of GPs. The White Paper does not describe how the movement towards greater equity will be achieved either. However, in December 1998 a revision to the payments received by doctors in deprived areas was announced following the 1998 report of the Doctors and Dentists Pay Review Body, which had recommended an increase in this payment. The higher payments are to go both to doctors working in deprived areas and to those developing new services for specific groups such as drug misusers and the elderly in nursing homes. Changes made to the Red Book (the rules governing general medical services) may also make it easier to recruit GPs in less popular areas, and many of the primary care pilots described by Clare Jenkins (see p.108) are in areas of deprivation. However, as Sir Donald Acheson's report notes, the impact of deprivation payments on the health of the most disadvantaged remains to be properly assessed.

The New NHS made clear the Government's aim of making more even the NHS's standard of care between different parts of the country. This intention was reaffirmed when, in March 1999, the guidelines on clinical governance were issued. In the words of the Secretary of State:

> *Patients have the right to expect that the same standards of care should be in place across the whole country. We want to tackle the unacceptable variations of service across the country, assuring quality and improving equity of access.*
>
> *We are introducing measures that will improve the quality of clinical services across the whole of the NHS. We have made clear our commitment to improving the poorer services, and making the good ones even better.*
> (PR 1999/0149)

The case for trying to even-up standards was illustrated by a 1999 report from the Stroke Association, *Stroke Care – A Matter of Chance*, which found, as its name implies, gaps in provision. Those admitted to hospitals in Wales, Scotland or Northern Ireland were found to be about twice as likely to be cared for in a stroke unit as patients admitted in England. It also found that about half of admissions were not managed in a stroke unit and access to neuro-imaging also varies a great deal. There was also a good deal of uncertainty among clinical staff as to what worked, which in turn was reflected in variations in the type of interventions used.

The measures set out in Part 1 of the Review, particularly Section 1.5, can be seen as trying to remove variations of this kind. But as we note there, the process is not likely to be equally successful everywhere. Furthermore, as the interim findings on the national service framework for coronary heart disease indicate, while there are some well-evidenced interventions that should be in general use, these alone do not define a single best pattern of provision. Hence a move towards a national standard may be premature. In practice, therefore, equality in the standard of provision may not yet be a sensible target, and indeed may never be as long as new forms of treatment and new evidence continue to emerge.

ACCESS

The high level performance indicators contain five indicators bearing on fair access, of which the first is a composite of age-standardised elective rates for:

- *CABG and PTCA*
- *hip replacement (aged 65 or over)*
- *knee replacement (aged 65 or over)*
- *cataract replacement.*

The notes to the indicators suggest that these are all procedures where there is considered to be substantial unmet need and that a lack of progress on this indicator may reflect inadequate commissioning plans or restricted capacity due to unexpected increases in emergency admissions.

The indicator itself does not reveal the underlying factors, i.e. whether they arise from the population itself, the primary care system or the hospital; neither can it show whether particular groups of the population are enjoying fair access.

Moreover, although this indicator embodies a number of very beneficial procedures, they represent only a small part of the elective care workload. As noted last year, the debate about waiting lists is curiously detached from the other objectives pursued by the NHS. The Government has set a national target for waiting list reduction, which has no significance from an equity perspective as it is not built up from local, equity-based targets, and it is pursuing the national target by rewarding those who do well in reducing the numbers waiting – which might make relative access worse.

As Anthony Harrison and Bill New argue elsewhere in this volume, from an equity viewpoint, a national target has no meaning; nor do waiting lists or times at local level unless they are specific to particular conditions or specialities. But such information is not available. That may explain why the second equity indicator is defined as (ii) *Size of in-patient waiting list per head of population (weighted)*.

The notes to the indicators suggest that the size of the waiting list per head of population illustrates where there are variations in supply and demand across the country. The waiting list per head of weighted population takes into account demographic differences between populations that affect the level of need for NHS care, but does not recognise other factors (such as those cited above) which might make for differences between them.

Furthermore, the Government has not directly addressed the critical issue – from an equity point of view – of prioritisation between patients and, hence, the time patients with different conditions have to wait. The Welsh Office, however, has done so – albeit on a trial basis. Its White Paper *NHS Wales: putting patients first*, published in January 1999, states that:

> *A more discriminating approach to waiting time is now needed – one which reconciles rising demand with available resources and which includes a greater emphasis on clinical prioritisation. This will provide quicker access to treatment for those who need it most.* (para.3.14)

This work remains exploratory and experimental but it is at least moving the debate in the right direction.

The third and fourth indicators are concerned with access to dentistry. They comprise *Adults registered with an NHS dentist* and *Children registered with an NHS dentist*.

As John Hayward notes, there are grounds for concern about access to NHS dentistry of a degree not matched by other services. These indicators should identify whether or not the situation is getting worse or whether the measures he describes are having an impact.

The fifth indicator is *Early detection of cancer*, a composite consisting of:

- *% of target population screened for breast cancer*
- *% of target population screened for cervical cancer.*

The notes suggest that this indicator can be used to assess the access of different socio-economic groups to disease prevention services, by comparing specific groups of health authorities, e.g. inner city health authorities against rural health authorities.

In 1999 the Cancer Research Campaign published *Cancer Research Campaign Cancer Stats (sic): Survival in England and Wales 1971–1995*, which showed that while for most cancers there was little difference between parts of Great Britain, there were statistically well-supported differences between the most affluent and the most deprived population groups. In some cases such as lung cancer these were small (though statistically significant) but for 16 adult cancers the difference was more than 5 per cent. According to the Executive Summary:

The 'gap' in survival between patients in the most affluent and most deprived groups was explored for the 41 cancers for which at least 1000 patients of known deprivation status were diagnosed during 1986–90. The difference in survival between patients in the most affluent and the most deprived groups exceeded 5% for sixteen adult cancers. A further twenty adult malignancies had a difference in five-year survival of between 0–5%, seven of which were statistically significant ... For some cancers the differences in survival between the most affluent and the most deprived groups are small (e.g. 1% for lung cancer) but the difference is still statistically significant due to the very large number of patients included in the survival estimates. (p.5)

Unfortunately, the analysis was unable to pinpoint the underlying factors: it simply goes on to say that possible explanations for lower survival in more deprived groups include:

longer delay in diagnosis or more advanced disease at diagnosis, worse general health or resistance to malignancy, different histological type of more aggressive disease, poorer access to optimal case and lower compliance with treatment. (p.5)

The wide spread of possibilities gives little indication of where to devote the effort to improve services to ensure the access criterion is met. Furthermore, other studies have found that delay in seeking diagnosis may be better explained by personal rather than social characteristics. The Government's Cancer Action Plan announced in May 1999 outlined a wide range of measures designed to improve cancer services, but it did not address the issue of where the need for improvement is greatest or whether a greater impact would be achieved by improving access. A commitment to making the NHS cancer services 'the best in the world' may, even if achieved, not result in a reduction in inequalities of outcome if the reasons for those lie outside the service itself.

The high level performance indicator set does not include access to GPs. However, it is one of the indicators proposed in the Treasury paper cited in Section 2.1. As noted above, the availability of GPs as measured by list size varies a great deal (see Table 2.3).

List size is in itself, even when weighted, an imperfect measure of relative access. For some time the Medical Practices Committee has been trying to improve the way it estimates the need for GPs but it has not found it easy to make progress. In 1997 it proposed a way of modifying simple list numbers as follows:

three high deprivation payments be counted as 1 notional patient;
four medium deprivation payments be counted as 1 notional patient; and
five low deprivation payments be counted as 1 notional patient.
(Medical Practices Committee Annual Report 1997/98, p.18)

TABLE 2.3

AVERAGE GP LIST SIZE BY NUMBER OF HAs

Average list size	*Number of HAs*
1600	4
1700	2
1750	11
1800	2
1850	8
1900	11
1950	15
2000	19
2050	15
2100	7
2150	5
2200	4
2250	1
2300	1

Source: Medical Practices Committee Annual Report 1997/98.

A system based on this adjustment, known as ALFRED, was introduced in 1998 and the MPC believes it has been useful in identifying practices 'which need extra medical commitment'. Its 1998 report adds that very few health authorities have used ALFRED to identify areas that need more doctors. The primary care pilots introduce further complexity since, in some cases, nurses are fulfilling what is currently a medical role. As this substitution grows, it will become more difficult to determine what an equitable distribution of medical resources is and, indeed, it becomes questionable if it is worthwhile, provided that financial resources are equalised satisfactorily.

OVERALL

Although the Government has made a commitment to reviewing the methods used to allocate financial resources to health authorities, this will not take effect until the next Comprehensive Spending Review. In the meantime, the Government, with the creation of the Modernisation Fund, has provided itself with a funding device that it can focus on whatever specific targets it wishes. The allocation of monies from this 'Fund' appears to be based on political and administrative judgement rather than systematic or widely applicable criteria. It is quite possible that these allocations will move the NHS away from equity rather than towards it.

So too may other elements of Government policy: the Secretary of State's commitment to improving the poorer services and making the good ones better may not result in a reduction in the disparity between services. As pointed out in Section 1.5, the drive towards equality of standards rests on over-simple assumptions as to the process of implementing the vast range of measures the Government is trying to introduce and the reasons why standards differ. In practice change cannot be uniform and standards of performance can never be equalised. Experience with GP fundholding and total purchasing suggests that primary care groups and primary care trusts (particularly the latter with their extensive freedoms) will develop at different rates and in different ways. Similarly, as Angela Coulter notes in her article, it will not be easy, even when the National Institute for Clinical Excellence is established, to eliminate all clinical variations.

These are practical considerations, but there is an issue of principle: in what services or circumstances should local choice predominate? In the case of waiting lists, Anthony Harrison and Bill New argue below that the national target is itself misconceived – not simply because it bears on numbers alone but because one total cannot reflect the situation across the NHS as a whole. Focusing on it may create greater differences between areas rather than the reverse. But it may well be appropriate for targets to be set for a narrow range of conditions where rapid access is critical, and to leave the rest to local choice.

Thus 'equal access for equal need' may not be the right objective, both for reasons of practice and principle. The NHS of course has always been diverse – and that diversity has given rise to the policies of the present Government. The points set out here suggest that limits as to how far this process can and should go must be acknowledged – but that would involve the centre (both Government and Executive) acknowledging limits to their ambitions. As of now, it seems unlikely that they will.

2.3 Accountability

The extension of accountability to clinical performance in the NHS is welcome, but how will the overall system function?

As we have seen in Section 1.1, the proposals being introduced as *The New NHS* is implemented are leading to a new 'map' of the NHS: new institutions and new roles have appeared, which in turn create new accountability requirements at local levels. At the same time, at the national level, the Treasury followed up the Comprehensive Spending Review with a White Paper, *Public Services for the Future: Modernisation, Reform, Accountability*, published in December 1998, which set an accountability framework for the public sector as a whole, comprising performance targets for each spending programme. Those for the Department of Health – omitting those relating to children in care – are in Box 2.2.

BOX 2.2: PERFORMANCE TARGETS FOR THE DEPARTMENT OF HEALTH

(i) Reduce premature deaths and avoidable illness, disease and injury, and reduce inequalities in health

(ii) Achieve the Government's commitment to reduce NHS inpatient waiting lists by 100,000 over the lifetime of the Parliament from the March 1997 position of 1.16 million, and deliver a consequential reduction in average waiting times

(iii) Ensure everyone with suspected cancer is able to see a specialist within two weeks of their GP deciding they need to be seen urgently and requesting an appointment: for all patients with suspected breast cancer by April 1999 and for all other cases of suspected cancer by 2000

(iv) Establish NHS Direct, so that everyone in England has access to a 24 hour telephone advice line staffed by nurses by December 2000

(v) Improve access to and quality of primary care services through investment in line with locally agreed Primary Care Investment Plans. Key targets are:
a) increase equity in the national distribution of GPs. From growth of approximately 0.6% whole-time-equivalent GPs in 1997 over 1996, there will be progress towards a national average annual increase of 1% whole-time-equivalent GPs by 2002, using a range of new initiatives and with local variations to take account of the need to concentrates on deprived and remote areas
b) increase investment in practice staff – 500 new practice nurses will be appointed by 2002
c) improve the quality of primary care premises, targeted towards areas of deprivation, resulting in improvements to 1000 premises nationally by 2002

(vi) Connect all GP surgeries which use clinical computer systems to the NHSnet by the end of 1999 and all other surgeries by the end of 2002, so that more information and services can be offered closer to people's homes

(vii) Improve the quality and effectiveness of treatment and care in the NHS by establishing the National Institute for Clinical Excellence by 1 April 1999, with a view to it producing at least 30 appraisals of new or existing technologies a year and guidance from 2000–01

(viii)Improve the responsiveness of NHS services by taking account of the views of patients and other users obtained through annual surveys of patient and user experience

(ix) Promote independence by reducing nationally the per capita rate of growth in emergency admissions of people aged over 75 to an annual average of 3% over the five years up to 2002–03, compared with an annual average rate of 3.5% over the last five years

(x) Improve the delivery of appropriate care and treatment to patients with mental illness who are discharged from hospital and reduce nationally the emergency psychiatric re-admission rate by 2 percentage points by 2002 from the 1998–98 baseline of 14.3%

(xi) Prevent the unnecessary loss of independence amongst older people by, as a first step, putting in place action plans in all local authorities, to be jointly agreed with the NHS and other local partners, covering prevention services, including respite care, by October 1999

Source: *Public services for the future: modernisation, reform, accountability: comprehensive spending review: public service agreements 1999–2002*. London: The Stationery Office, 1998, pp.3–4.

The White Paper was followed up by a Treasury consultation paper in March 1999, *The Government's Measures of Success: output and performances analyses*, which set out for each Department a series of objectives and measures similar to those cited above, together with a list of performance measures, which we have drawn on in the previous Section.

In principle, Departments will lose money if they fail to perform, turning them, in the words of Sir Peter Kemp, a former Permanent Secretary, into area managers for the Treasury. How that could be done in practice is hard to see – unless of course the Treasury was prepared to set up a shadow department to which the money would be transferred to see if it could do better.

The Department of Health, as we noted last year, published proposals for a national performance assessment framework, which set out criteria under six headings by which the performance of its 'area' would be judged. As a result of the consultation on the paper issued in January 1998, a number of changes were made to the proposed list of 'high level' indicators, from which we have already drawn in this Review.

In April 1999, *The NHS Performance Assessment Framework* (HSC 1999/078) was published setting out how the framework should work. The Circular sets out the way in which the framework is to be used in the form of a simple diagram (see Figure 2.1).

It states that:

> *Over time, the Framework will have an important role in the formal accountability arrangements of the NHS, to ensure that all the organisations in health communities are playing their part in working to improve performance across the six areas of the Framework, including:*
>
> - *the* ***Health Improvement Programme****, which will identify targets for measurable improvements in health and health care.*
> - ***Annual accountability arrangements*** *between a Health Authority and its local Primary Care Groups which will contain key*

FIGURE 2.1

ACCOUNTABILITY ARRANGEMENTS IN THE NEW NHS

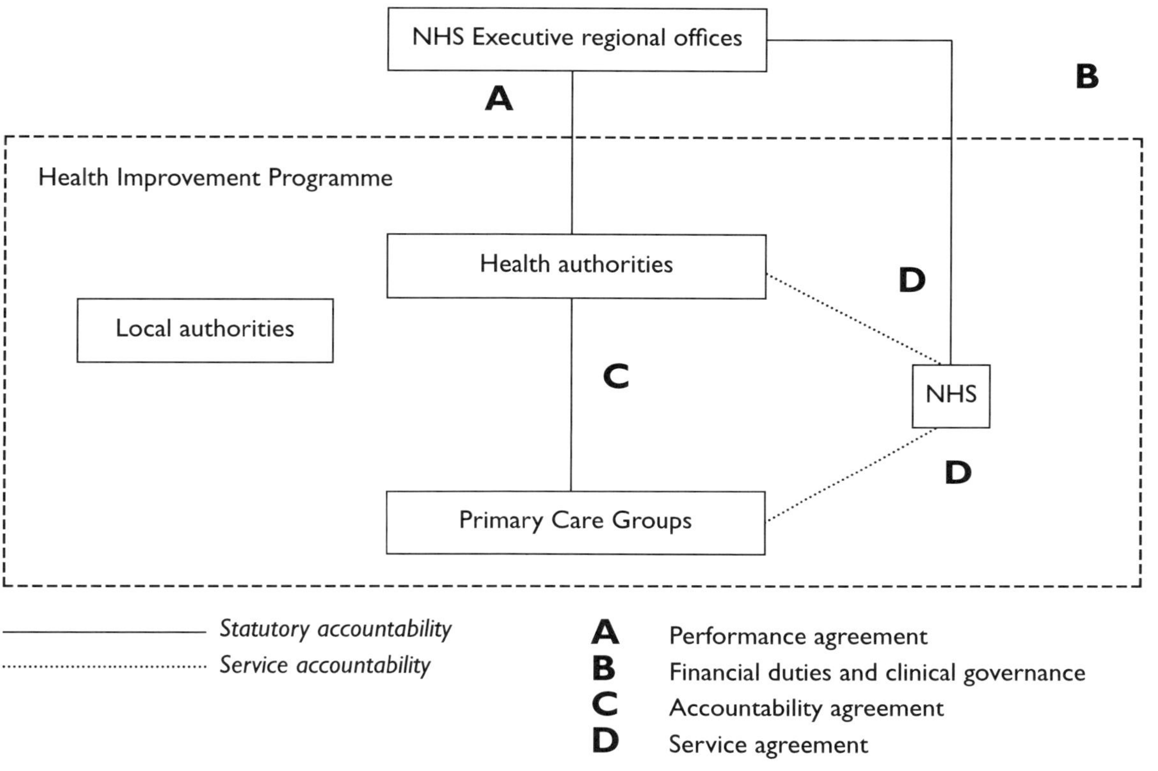

targets, objectives and standards for the provision or commissioning of services.

- ***Service agreements** between Health Authorities/Primary Care Groups and NHS Trusts which will be patient/service based and developed typically at Clinical Directorate level.*
- *NHS Executive Regional Offices and the Regional Offices of the Social Services Inspectorate, which will continue to monitor jointly performance across the **NHS/Social care interface**.*
- *Each HA working with its Regional Office to develop an annual **performance agreement** covering all the key objectives of the HA for the year.* (HSC 1999/078, pp.13–14)

The document does not make clear, however, what the links should be between these indicators, the clinical indicators described in Section 1.5 and the targets set out in the Treasury paper. In the case of the target for GPs, for example, the Government itself has a prime role through its control of deprivation payments; the General Practices Committee retains the prime responsibility for the distribution of GPs; the NHS Executive authorises the PMS pilots described in Section 1.1; and health authorities and, in time, primary care trusts may also have a part to play.

More generally, although the Figure shows a single line combining financial duties and clinical governance, it does not clarify what the relationship between the two should be. We noted in Section 1.5 that the steps taken to introduce clinical governance and improve service quality are independent of finance. On the financial side, the system of controls assurance described in previous Health Policy Reviews has been further developed, but this too does not make the link across the other way, to quality.

In March 1999, *Corporate Governance in the NHS: controls assurance statements* (HSC 1999/070) set out the next steps in the introduction of controls assurance statements for NHS trusts and health authorities. After setting out some points to be covered for the 1998/99 accounts, it goes on to set out the more comprehensive requirements for 1999/2000. In particular:

> *An organisation's ability to make a sensible assurance statement will be built upon a soundly-based risk management strategy. From 1999/2000, every Health Authority and NHS Trust will be required to have such a strategy containing the following elements:*
> - *the continuous identification and prioritisation of key risks;*
> - *a description of actions taken to manage each key risk; and*
> - *the identification of how risk is measured.*
>
> *The information that flows from the above needs to be:*
> - *relevant and understandable;*
> - *forward-looking in its perspective;*
> - *suitable for the range of intended audiences;*
> - *clear regarding timescales involved; and*
> - *in accord with patient and other confidentiality requirements.* (HSC 1999/070, para.11)

Subsequently *Governance in the New NHS: controls assurance statement 1999/2000 risk management and operational controls* (HSC 1999/123, 21 May 1999) expanded on these requirements to include the following:

> *ensure that the appropriate structures are in place within their organisation for implementing controls assurance taking account of linkages with clinical governance and, where applicable, NHS risk pooling schemes;*
> *from October 1999, conduct a baseline self-assessment of compliance with risk management and organisational controls standards;*
> *formulate a prioritised action plan with clearly assigned responsibilities in the light of this assessment;*
> *provide an assurance statement within their Annual Report for 1999/2000; and*
> *ensure appropriate arrangements are in place to verify the assurance statement.* (HSC 1999/123, p.2)

As the Circular indicates, these measures are to be seen in the context of clinical governance. The overall picture is set out in Figure 2.2 as follows:

FIGURE 2.2

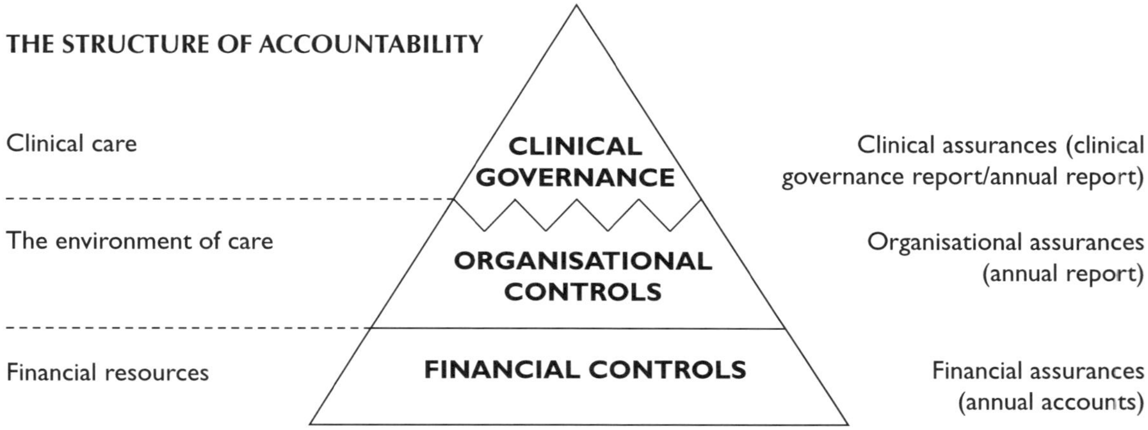

The assurance statements are intended to bring a series of benefits:

- *reduction in risk exposure through more effective targeting of resources to address key risk areas;*
- *improvements in economy, efficiency and effectiveness resulting from a reduction in the frequency and/or severity of incidents, complaints, claims, staff absence and other loss;*
- *demonstrable compliance with applicable laws and regulations;*
- *enhanced reputation through public disclosure of achievements in meeting objectives and managing risk; and, consequently,*
- *increased public confidence in the quality of services provided by the NHS.* (HSC 1999/123, p.4)

The arrangements for clinical governance set out in *Clinical Governance in the New NHS* (HSC 1999/065, 16 March 1999) state that 'reports to the Board' will be an important part of the accountability mechanisms that underpin clinical governance. However, what these reports should contain is still to be defined and how, if at all, they should be related to the financial reports that will continue to be necessary remains to be elucidated.

Figure 2.2 suggests that the controls assurance statements are intended to 'underpin' clinical governance but, in fact, although the procedures of clinical governance may be separate from finance, decisions as to how to provide services are not. Thus although the Figure suggests a close link between finance and clinical performance, the nature of that link, and at what levels in each trust it should be made, are yet to be determined.

While these developments were designed to tighten internal controls over finance and clinical activity, the new organisations created by the implementation of *The New NHS* raise different issues. The creation of primary care groups marks the beginning of a process that will transfer responsibility for spending decisions away from health authorities. The arrangements for GP fundholding were widely held to be inadequate; accordingly, those for primary care groups, set out in *The New NHS Modern and Dependable Developing Primary Care Groups* (HSC 1998/139, 30 August 1998), are more elaborate. The Circular states that:

> *29. As a committee of the Health Authority, the Primary Care Group Board will be accountable through its Chair to the Chief Executive of the Health Authority. The establishment of Primary Care Groups does not diminish the Health Authority Chief Executive's responsibilities for ensuring both propriety and value for money in the use of public funds.* (HSC 1998/139, p.12)

It goes on:

> *36. The relationship between the Health Authority and Primary Care Groups will be expressed in an* ***annual accountability agreement****. This will contain key targets, objectives and standards for the delivery or commissioning of services. The agreement will also be the vehicle for setting out the Group's Primary Care Investment Plan. Progress will be monitored against this agreement. It will need to be consistent with national priorities and the local Health Improvement Programme and should be expressed in such a way as to be monitored in line with the Performance Assessment Framework for the NHS. The annual accountability agreement should not become a bureaucratic document but should be relevant to the aims and objectives agreed between the Health Authority and the Primary Care Group.* (HSC 1998/139, p.14)

At the same time, the groups are required to:

- *have open and transparent processes (including open meetings) to allow stakeholders and the public to see the basis upon which Primary Care Groups take decisions*
- *have regular communications with stakeholders to inform and disseminate their decisions*
- *produce annual accountability agreements setting out their plans and reflecting on their*

outturn performance. These will be public documents available through the Health Authority

- *have clear and open clinical governance arrangements to enable stakeholders to develop confidence in the operation of the Group.* (HSC 1998/139, p.14)

These requirements will, like the other tasks that PCGs are required to perform, be demanding in terms of commitment of time and other resources – both for the groups themselves and health authorities.

If and when primary care groups develop into primary care trusts, further issues will arise. One of the main purposes in establishing a free-standing primary care trust is to give it more freedom of manoeuvre than a primary care group has as a committee of a health authority. Such freedom, precisely because it may be misused, requires additional accountability arrangements in what up to now has been a relatively unaccountable corner of the NHS.

The broad arrangements for primary care trusts are set out in Box 2.3. In the words of *Primary Care Trusts*:

> *Unless there are particular difficulties within the Primary Care Trust, the role of the Health Authority should be one of monitoring overall performance rather than direction or day-to-day involvement. It will be for the Primary Care Trust to decide how best to meet the needs of its population within this framework. The Secretary of State will retain similar reserve powers to those he holds for all NHS bodies to take action, if necessary.*

However, it recognises that the freedom the trusts will enjoy entails risks – in particular the aim of putting doctors, nurses and other health care professionals in the 'driving seat' as the executives of the trust (though not of the board) may give rise to actual or perceived conflicts of interest. For example, decisions on the type of services to be provided could be seen to favour one group over another.

BOX 2.3: ACCOUNTABILITY FOR PRIMARY CARE TRUSTS

Primary care trusts will be a key part of the NHS. Like other NHS bodies they will need to be accountable at a number of levels:

- nationally to the Secretary of State and by working within national policy frameworks, including guidance on national priorities
- locally to the health authority, the health improvement programme, the public and the wider body of professionals in the area they serve.

Accountability to the health authority

A primary care trust will be accountable to its health authority (and, as with all other NHS bodies, to the Secretary of State) by means of an annual accountability agreement, which will spell out agreed aims and targets for improving health, health services and value for money.

Accountability to the public

Primary care trusts will also have a wider accountability to the public and to the wider body of professionals in the area they serve. Local accountability to the public will be exercised formally through:

- the lay members of the board
- public board meetings and an annual published report
- complaints procedures which mirror those of health authorities for commissioning activities, and NHS trusts for direct service provision – including being within the remit of the Parliamentary Commissioner for Administration
- relationships with the community health council on a par with health authorities for commissioning activities, and with NHS trusts for direct service provision.

Source: *Primary Care Trusts*. London: Department of Health, 1999, p.15.

BOX 2.4: THE PUBLIC AUDIT FORUM

The four national agencies, the National Audit Office, the Northern Ireland Audit Office, the Audit Commission for Local Authorities and the National Health Service in England and Wales, and the Accounts Commission for Scotland, have established the Public Audit Forum to provide a focus for developmental thinking in relation to public audit. The main role of the Forum is consultative and advisory. It is not able to direct the national audit agencies and other bodies involved in public audit.

Specific elements of the Forum's remit are to:

- provide a strategic focus on issues cutting across the work of the national audit agencies
- build visibly on the existing co-operation between the national audit agencies to enhance the efficiency and effectiveness of public audit, whilst, in all matters, respecting the statutorily and constitutionally independent status of the agencies in the selection, execution and reporting of their work and in determining how this work should be organised and staffed
- establish definitions of what constitutes public audit in so far as this differs from and goes beyond the current interpretation of company audit
- advise on the application of standards and the practices of the auditors of bodies delivering public services, including on the quality of service to be provided to such audited bodies, having regard to the statements issued by the Auditing Practices Board
- develop standards for use by auditors of bodies delivering public services where none have been issued by the Auditing Practices Board
- advise on the resolution of common technical problems and disseminate good and innovative practice in tackling common issues
- provide the considered view of the national audit agencies on any developments or proposals which impact on public audit, whilst avoiding comment on the merits of Government policy objectives.

Source: www.public-audit-forum.gov.uk/about.htm

As noted in Section 2.2, while these proposals bear on the way individual parts of the NHS should operate, the Government's emphasis on co-operation across organisational boundaries poses new issues for accountability. The nature of these issues was put clearly in a paper from the Public Audit Forum (see Box 2.4) issued in April 1999.

It points out that public services are increasingly being delivered by charitable, voluntary and private organisations and that, as a result, the lines of accountability to Parliament are being blurred. Furthermore, in some areas, there is joint responsibility within the public sector for some spending programmes, with the result that one part of the public sector may be responsible for finance and another for delivery.

The existing monitoring and audit processes are ill adapted to these new requirements. There are examples of joint working – for example the joint reviews of social services conducted by the Audit Commission and the Social Services Inspectorate – but these are the exceptions that prove the rule. There are no regularly collected data series or audit procedures which 'follow the patient' across different parts of the NHS, let alone the NHS and other care providers.

The high level performance indicators include four indicators that bear on performance at the health/social care interface:

- discharge from hospital
- delayed discharge from hospital for people aged 75 or over

- emergency psychiatric re-admission rate
- emergency admissions to hospital for people aged 75 and over

But while these are of value in pinpointing possible weaknesses, they do not in themselves shed light on why things went wrong and hence cannot attribute responsibility. What that process should be remains unclear.

THE PUBLIC AT LARGE

We noted above some of the first results of the National User Survey. In announcing its plans for cancer care, the Government indicated that it intended to survey users of cancer services. We also noted above the interim monitoring results for NHS Direct and the Government's proposals for expert patients.

These developments, while not forming part of the formal apparatus of accountability, are clearly welcome. But what remains unclear is how they fit into the arrangements set out above. The figures above have no place for those who use the NHS but, as the National User Surveys become more specific, the surveys will almost certainly reveal that particular aspects of the Service are seen as being poorly or inappropriately delivered or will identify specific gaps. In the case of social care, for example, users continue to complain that they are not offered what they want, i.e. help with housework rather than personal care, and that many aspects of the quality of what they are offered is not satisfactory. Equally, well-informed patients may well choose a different course of action to that recommended by professionals. If they do so, then, provided that they have been appropriately advised, responsibility lies with the patient and the nature of professional accountability must be modified.

The Government came to power pledged to introduce a Freedom of Information Act. A draft Bill was published in May 1999, and was widely criticised on the grounds that it would prove much more restrictive than what had been originally intended. In November 1998, however, the Government had published *Opening up NHS Board Meetings to the Public* (HSC1998/207), which stated that the 'Government is committed to ending what it sees as excessive secrecy in decision-making in public bodies'.

The Circular sets out in some detail what it regards as good practice in relation to physical access, timing and location of meetings, and similar matters. It also notes the intention to bring primary care groups within the scope of the legislation. It would seem that the Government is keener to open up the workings of the organisations for which it is responsible than it is to reveal its own functions.

OVERALL

It has been remarked that the NHS is the most scrutinised organisation in the UK. The innovations set out here seem set to increase rather than diminish its exposure. Given its nature as a public service, that may appear to be an unmitigated good, particularly where, as with clinical governance, a gaping hole in existing arrangements around the core business of the NHS – delivering care – seems set to be filled. Although the process of implementing clinical governance will be slow, it is hardly contentious to expect that the gap should be plugged in time and, in particular, that better arrangements should be in place for dealing with poor performance by individual clinicians and institutions. Similarly, as long as the Secretary of State purports to account for the Service to Parliament, it seems appropriate that he should have available the information needed to judge whether it is performing well.

But while the extension of effective accountability in this sense is welcome, it is hard to see how the overall system will function. In part this is a matter of knowledge and technique. As we have pointed out in Sections 2.1 and 2.2, the interpretation of the indicators in the performance framework is far from straightforward and, as we noted in relation to cancer care, where differences are found it may be impossible to determine their origins.

This difficulty is compounded by the nature of the 'new NHS'. In the case of the failures in the screening programme at the Kent and Canterbury Trust (see *Health Care UK 1997/98*), the Government attributed the shortcoming identified there to the competitive and divisive nature of the *ancien régime*. But the *nouveau régime* may in fact have greater weaknesses from the standpoint of accountability. In the case of cancer care, where a national framework is almost in place, the Government has supported the developed of a system of care running across the existing units of accountability – NHS trusts – leaving open the question of how the interfaces between them are to be handled. When the Commission for Health Improvement comes to investigate how this system is working, it may find it hard, if weaknesses are identified, to decide whether to attribute them to individual clinicians, their organisations or the financial framework within which they work.

In particular, the emphasis on co-operation and joint working means that failure to perform cannot be simply attributed to any one organisation. For example, the means to achieve a reduction in emergency admissions lie with different bodies and because the value of any action taken depends on what others do, no simple attribution of 'blame' may be possible. Furthermore, in respect of continuing care, non-NHS organisations that fall outside the proposed lines of accountability altogether may be involved. The logic of the concern with clinical performance should have led to a unified system of regulation running across public, private and voluntary providers. Instead, as we noted in Sections 1.3 and 1.5, separate systems are proposed.

While this point is primarily one for the public sector professionals, it also applies to individuals. Those seeking redress through the Ombudsman are faced with the choice of going to the Health or to the Local Government Ombudsman if they have a complaint arising from a mishandled discharge from hospital. As pointed out in Section 1.5, there is an obvious case for unification or joint jurisdiction, just as there is for the uniform arrangements across the public and the private sector.

Finally, as the ambitions of the centre grow, the risk that central and local targets will conflict also increases. These conflicts may arise through the incompatible requirements of managerial time and financial and clinical resources, and also through linkages between different parts of the health (and social) care sector that have been ignored centrally or which, like the twin pressures on hospital beds of elective and emergency care, can only be reconciled in the light of detailed local knowledge. The central difficulty here is that the Government cannot 'performance manage' the whole of the NHS but equally, as things currently stand, it cannot create genuinely independent local 'NHSs' with their own lines of accountability. Short of major devolution within England, that dilemma cannot be resolved.

Part 3 Calendar of Events

SEPTEMBER 1998

9 **Pay:** £1000 pay boost announced for nurses, midwives and professions allied to medicine.

10 **Screening:** £2.5 million pilot scheme for screening bowel cancer announced.

14 **Viagra:** doctors advised not to prescribe Viagra at NHS expense until further notice.

23 **Public health:** programme to encourage and enable young people to participate more in physical activity announced.

24 **Information technology:** *Information for Health*, a £1 billion modernisation of NHS IT systems announced.

29 **National booked admissions programme:** £25 million investment in pilots for instant booking system.

A&E services: one in four departments to be modernised.

30 **Waiting lists:** Secretary of State announces extra £320 million to keep waiting lists falling.

Beacon awards: NHS to invest £10 million a year in identifying and promoting 100 beacon local health services to reward and spread best practice.

Hospital beds: Secretary of State sets up national beds inquiry.

OCTOBER 1998

7 **Primary care:** £5 million announced for second wave Personal Medical Services pilots.

Waiting lists: further fall in numbers on in-patient waiting lists announced.

8 **National Survey of Patients Views:** first national survey announced.

15 **NHS Direct:** Government introduces plans for a single telephone number for the whole country, to be available nationally in the year 2000.

NOVEMBER 1998

2 **Costs:** Reference cost tables published revealing huge cost differences between hospitals.

3 **Winter planning:** Secretary of State announces extra £250 million for the NHS to prevent a winter crisis.

4 **Waiting lists:** figures for end of September 1998 published, showing the largest monthly decrease recorded.

10 **Finance:** cash allocations for health authorities published.

Information technology: the first 'PRODIGY' system launched, giving prescribing advice to GPs while they see their patients.

26 **Health inequalities:** Acheson report into health inequalities published.

27 **Legislation:** Road Traffic (NHS Charges) Bill published.

30 **Social Services:** White Paper *Modernising Social Services* published.

DECEMBER 1998

2 **Waiting lists:** monthly figures show fall for six consecutive months.

9 **Public health:** White Paper *Smoking Kills* published, setting out Government plans to reduce smoking.

10 **Pay:** pay boost announced for GPs in poorest areas.

28 **Waiting lists:** NHS trusts to be rewarded for making good progress in reducing waiting lists by benefiting from share in £32 million performance fund.

JANUARY 1999

13 **Public health:** review of the National Air Quality Strategy published by the Department of the Environment.

Emergency care: joint call centres for fire, police and ambulance services to be piloted.

19 **Dentistry:** funding announced for a second wave of Personal Dental Service pilots.

Health inequalities: Sure Start programme announced to help 60 disadvantaged areas of the country to increase opportunity and create equal chances for all children.

20 **Health Action Zones:** £78 million investment funding for first and second wave Zones announced.

21 **Viagra:** six-week public consultation on prescription of the drug announced by the Secretary of State.

25 **Public health:** Smoking Control Network launched.

FEBRUARY 1999

1 **Pay:** Pay Review Body awards met in full.

2 **Mental health:** £84 million over three years allocated to improve mental health services for children.

NHS Direct: Government unveils plans to extend the scheme to cover 60 per cent of the population by the end of 1999.

3 **National Institute for Clinical Excellence:** consultation proposals published on how the new organisation will operate.

4 **Fraud:** Government tightens up on home visits by mobile optical practices.

8 **Carers:** National Strategy for Carers published.

13 **Finance:** Prime Minister announces the modernisation of one in three A&E departments with an extra £30 million.

15 **Pay:** Secretary of State announces radical plans to modernise the NHS pay structure.

20 **Primary care:** discussion paper on primary care trusts published.

21 **Waiting lists:** £20 million extra allocated for equipment and facilities to reduce waiting lists.

Long-term care: Health Committee report into long-term care published.

22 **Social services:** consultation paper on performance tables for social services published.

MARCH 1999

1 **Long-term care:** *With Respect to Age* report of Royal Commission on Long-term Care published.

2 **Waiting lists:** number of people on waiting lists lower than any time since March 1997.

3 **Hospital buildings:** details given of a £1.1 billion capital investment in hospital buildings, including plans to end mixed-sex accommodation.

5 **Cancer services:** £10 million allocated to improve lung cancer services.

9 **Public health:** Healthy Workplace Initiative launched.

Public health: Chancellor announces 5 per cent rise in tax on tobacco in budget.

10 **Legislation:** Road Traffic Accidents (NHS Funding) Bill receives Royal Assent.

14 **A&E services:** all departments to be modernised.

Cancer services: £150 million made available from National Lottery for cancer services.

22 **Information technology:** primary care groups awarded £20 million to be targeted at upgrading their IT systems.

23 **Public health:** first ever Government strategy on sexual health announced.

26 **Fraud:** new fraud strategy announced, 'Countering fraud in the NHS'.

30 **Waiting lists:** target reduction of 100,000 met one month early.

Public health: plan of action set in place to tackle obesity.

APRIL 1999

1 **Cancer:** two weeks breast cancer target met.

Charges: free eye tests for the over 60s and prescription charges raised by 20p – the lowest amount for 20 years.

11 **National Survey of Patient's Views:** initial results published.

12 **Walk-in centres:** £20 million allocated from the Modernisation Fund to create 20 NHS fast access walk-in centres.

16 **NHS Direct:** third wave of sites announced.

Public health: smoking cessation services to be provided by the NHS.

20 **General practice research database:** allocated £3 million for investment and management by Medicines' Control Agency.

National services framework: work begins on framework for diabetes.

23 **Health Action Zones:** 15 new Zones created in second round of pilots.

27 **Public health:** National Heart Forum report on coronary heart disease prevention published.

29 **Fraud:** £3 million investment allocated to new counter-fraud operational service.

Paediatric care: £15 million allocated to children's intensive care.

MAY 1999

7 **Viagra:** results of consultation published and final decision announced on eligibility.

Capital investment strategy: first ever publication of capital strategy for NHS and social services.

10 **Public health:** publication of a guide for health care professionals on how to help people stop smoking.

Waiting lists: Government announces largest fall in numbers on waiting lists yet.

20 **Cancer services:** Prime Minister announces a 10-year cancer action plan to save 60,000 lives at the 'cancer summit'.

21 **Doctors:** new agreement on junior doctors' hours announced.

27 **Dentistry:** funding announced for second wave of Personal Dental Services pilots.

JUNE 1999

4 **Waiting lists:** numbers on waiting lists show rise in April.

7 **Carers:** 'Caring for Carers' award launched for those who care for relatives, friends and family and those who support them.

10 **Public health:** two independent studies find no link between the MMR vaccine and autism.

15 **Private health care:** consultation document 'Regulating Private and Voluntary Healthcare' published.

16 **Clinical performance:** publication of first set of clinical indicators and high level performance indicators.

21 **Doctors:** 1000 additional undergraduate medical places announced.

22 **Funding:** £2.5 million to be invested in patient consultation programme, Health in Partnership.

23 **Professional boards:** the creation of three new professional boards to regulate speech therapists, clinical scientists and paramedics was announced.

Cancer: new cancer beacons, services of excellence across the country to be identified.

24 **Procurement:** Cabinet Office review into NHS purchasing published.

30 **Legislation:** Health Act receives Royal assent.

JULY 1999

6 **Public health:** White Paper, *Saving Lives: Our Healthier Nation* published.

Waiting lists: figures show a slight rise in May.

7 **NHS Direct:** data published shows that a quarter of a million patients have been helped since the telephone line's launch.

9 **Nursing:** new nursing strategy 'Making a Difference' introduced by Prime Minister and Secretary of State.

13 **Pharmaceutical costs:** new pharmaceutical price regulation scheme agreement announced, aimed to cut branded drug costs by 4.5 per cent.

15 **Long-term care:** Health Select Committees report published.

16 **Primary care:** third wave of primary care pilots announced.

19 **Mental health:** consultation document *Managing people with severe personality disorder* published by Home Office and Department of Health.

POLICY NOTES

Emerging problems with merger policy

There is strong pressure from the centre for more mergers in the NHS: new measures are needed to prevent mergers causing more problems than they solve.

John McClenahan

Mergers in the NHS are currently all the rage. Trust merging with trust, health authority with health authority, combining practices into PCGs, and service rationalisation between sites all have similar effects. In this and the previous financial year, around 100 trusts in England alone were or will be involved in mergers – over one-fifth of the total[1] – and there are similar developments in Wales and Scotland.

In supporting mergers the Government might be hoping to realise:

- reduced management costs
- improved quality of service, resulting from (for example) better out-of-hours medical cover, co-located clinical teams, or better sited facilities
- improved ability to deliver strategic service change through bringing different 'factions' under one organisational and management umbrella.

As far as we are aware, these possible merger aims are not clearly spelled out in Government policy documents. Despite the strong pressure behind these developments, the Department of Health has not made clear the rationale for the specific mergers it appears to support, other than to claim substantial management cost savings and the benefits of service rationalisation. But in doing so it has not made clear how in practice these might be achieved; nor has it paid proper attention to the downside risks of poorly conducted mergers, such as loss of staff morale and a lower level of organisational performance.

These risks are considerable. Much of the available evidence suggests that the anticipated benefits of merger are rarely achieved in practice, and the underlying rationale for seeking a merger is often both unclear and unlikely to succeed.[2]

Several recent publications have expressed variants of this message. Goddard and Ferguson have concluded that the economic benefits of mergers are modest at best.[3] The present author and colleagues, summarising the work of others on the impact of mergers on staff health, found that organisational performance always suffers in the short-term and there can be severe impacts on the mental and physical health of staff.[4]

Cost savings from management overhead reduction are small even in anticipation, typically estimated at £200–300,000 per annum or less than 1 per cent of the total budgets of the combined organisations.[3] Furthermore, these savings are usually outweighed in reality by a combination of the unanticipated direct costs of supporting the merger process and the unmeasured, but often substantial, loss of morale and productivity for several years resulting from disrupted relationships and communication patterns, and increased stress from fear of job loss, forced change of location or role reassignment. This latter loss is found even in the most successful mergers.[1]

If NHS management costs are *forced* to reduce quickly, the savings are even more likely to be offset by these hidden but nonetheless real losses in the actual performance of the combined operation.

Given that the political pressure supporting mergers may be irresistible, or the path to merger has already been embarked upon, what policy implications are there for central government? And what can the leaders of health care organisations do to minimise the damaging impacts that are almost always felt in the short-term? How can Health Service mergers improve on the likelihood of success from the typically reported 15–20 per cent of all private sector mergers?[2]

To answer these questions it is useful to think of four stages in a merger:

- pre-merger
- the merger itself – around and shortly after the time of formal combination
- post-merger
- long-term 'living together'.

How people are treated and how they respond to change matters at all stages, but the issues vary over time, between different staff groups, and in the different sites and organisations involved.

At least two years are needed following mergers for the benefits to be realised, and it can take longer,[1] even when the merger is a 'success'. One study of 100 major organisational changes – not mergers but on a similar scale – suggested that it took five years for the most important changes to be achieved.[5] It follows that if mergers are to produce benefits, they must be planned and implemented with this long-term horizon in mind.

In practice, however, most management attention is typically focused as follows: in pre-merger discussions on financial issues; at merger time on the local politics of the situation; and post-merger on limiting the damage that is by then often apparent. The longer-term requirements of success tend to be ignored.

This is also true of central government, which has followed the typical pattern of focusing on the anticipated financial benefits of merger, or seeing them as the only way to secure strategic service delivery change. Government has additionally emphasised meeting trade union concerns of job losses or worsening employment conditions through support for TUPE.

Overall, there has been too much emphasis on stage one – pre-merger discussion – and, as has been the pattern in other contexts, the Government has typically focused on the expected savings and other benefits and has *not* paid real attention to the crucial issue of how *people* are handled and motivated throughout *all* the stages of merger over a long period.

Against this background it is not surprising that early examples of the results of NHS mergers are not encouraging. For example, recent reports suggest that the savings of over £4 million per annum expected from merging Barnet and Edgware trusts (and their acute hospitals) in north London have not been achieved, and are unlikely to be achieved.[6]

As part of their recent review of mergers, the HEA invited comment from the NHS about senior staff's experience of merger. Only a few respondents indicated that they felt their local merger had been well-executed (e.g. Pinderfields and Pontefract), and even they felt (in common with research experience from outside the NHS) that it would be some years before major benefits are realised.

Poorly executed mergers, or ones with poorly explained or frankly disbelieved aims, are among several factors damaging the morale of the very people who are key to making them successful. Senior clinical staff, particularly consultants, are seriously disenchanted with the merger process.

A high proportion of NHS consultants attending recent King's Fund programmes are so thoroughly disillusioned by what they *perceive* (rightly or wrongly) as broken central government promises that they have almost opted out of engagement in service redesign following merger. It is not that they do not support the policy intentions, but rather that they do not see how to make a constructive input in the face of so many contradictory central demands – to reorganise the merged service, shorten waiting lists, reduce junior doctors' hours, provide a more consumer-responsive service, make better use of research evidence, protect time for teaching and research, and liaise more closely with primary care – while still seeing more patients personally, keeping their technical skills up-to-date, and making do with fewer supporting staff in the interests of increased 'efficiency'. They are not even receiving much from the increase in consultant numbers promised by successive governments, and are mistrustful of past failures to anticipate training needs in key specialties such as obstetrics and gynaecology, anaesthetics and oncology. Their experience of the reality of policy implementation is flatly contradictory to other Government 'commitments' to making the NHS a better place to work.

It is easy to dismiss this as 'whinging' or looking for someone else to blame, but the reality of pressure in consultants' working lives as they describe it in confidential discussion groups cannot be denied. They are key to making many of the proposed changes work, yet have felt forced to adopt a cynical attitude to centrally driven policy initiatives as a defence mechanism against perpetual work overload in what is, at best, an inherently stressful job. It does not help that a workaholic culture has become endemic in the senior NHS management level, as in so many other parts of the economy.

It is not so much that the 'pace of change' should slow, as that the practical consequences of the pressures to merge (along with other hotly pursued policy changes) should be better recognised centrally. Achieving change is not free of cost or effort, yet the expressed intention is usually that it should be done within existing and already tight 'envelopes' of money and time.

Some parts of the NHSE and its regional offices are offering practical help, training and development, or resources to support change – and this is welcomed by those involved in implementing change. However, the efforts are perceived as too limited in the face of the massive change agenda facing senior and middle clinical and management staff, and not backed in reality by Government resources, as opposed to intention and exhortation.

The Health Education Authority has attempted work in this field, and recently published guidance aimed at board members and senior NHS managers and clinical staff on minimising the negative impact of mergers on staff health. This advice includes more general observations and suggestions for improving the merger process (see Box 1).

BOX 1: MERGERS: HEALTH EDUCATION AUTHORITY ADVICE

Pre-merger
- clarifying the *real* reasons for merger locally
- exploring the cultural as well as strategic fit between the merging organisations

At merger
- giving serious forethought to the *process* of making the merger work
- providing clear, open and honest two-way communication to convey the reasons for merger; the likely timetable of the process; and how jobs and career prospects may be affected
- involving the HR department and its expertise early on
- recognising that what you *do* matters more than what you *say* – 'actions speak louder than words' – and that early actions have great symbolic as well as literal significance to anxious staff

Post-merger
- making the actions taken post-merger consistent with the declared values and aims of the merger, avoiding internal contradictions (for example, not appointing to all the top posts from just one organisation, if this was declared to be a partnership making the best of both pre-merger worlds)
- taking key decisions speedily to minimise anxiety and uncertainty – especially about filling the top posts – and publishing and maintaining a timetable of when other decisions will be made
- sustaining attention to, and actively supporting and resourcing, the merger process for a long time after the merger, and not just focusing on delivering promised results (which are unlikely to be achieved if the process is neglected)
- actively supporting the most vulnerable staff groups – middle managers and clinical staff, staff in departments targeted for cost savings, and top managers whose jobs or roles are threatened

Source: adapted from McClenahan *et al. Healthy Ever After? Supporting staff through merger and beyond*. HEA, 1999.

If mergers are going to succeed the Government should consider:

- clarifying the real reasons underpinning the political thrust for merger, and tailoring the general argument to particular mergers
- resourcing adequate organisational development support for the organisations and individuals most involved in mergers
- matching actions more closely to intentions to reduce cynicism amongst key staff groups whose support will be crucial in realising the intended benefits.

If these steps are taken, then mergers in future may have a reasonable chance of success.

REFERENCES

1. Crail M. Bitter pill: forty-nine trusts working towards merger. *Health Services Journal* 1999; 109 (5638): 10–11.

2. Cartwright S and Cooper CL. The human effects of mergers and acquisitions. In: Cooper CL and Rousseau DM, editors. *Trends in organisational behaviour*. Chichester: John Wiley and Sons Ltd, 1994: Vol. 1.

3. Goddard M and Ferguson B. Mergers in the NHS: made in heaven or marriages of convenience? *Nuffield occasional papers Health Economics series*. London: Nuffield Trust, 1996: Paper No. 1.

4. McClenahan JW, Howard L and Macknight A. *Healthy Ever After? Supporting staff through merger and beyond*. London: Health Education Authority, 1999.

5. Kotter JP. Why transformation efforts fail. *Harvard Business Review* 1995; 73: 2.

6. Whitfield L. Sorry is the hardest word. *Health Services Journal* 1998; 108: 16.

NHS dentistry

NHS dental provision has changed significantly in the last decade – and not always for the better. A clear long-term view of its place in the NHS is required to prevent the decline of NHS dentistry.

John Hayward

Over the last ten years there have been significant changes in NHS dentistry, including revisions to the dental contract for NHS work, changes in the system of remuneration and changes in patient registration periods. Evidence has also accumulated to reinforce anecdotal concerns of not only reduced access to NHS dental care, but also declines in the dental health of some sections of the population.

Policy objectives for NHS dentistry have not, however, been clear; nor do they, apparently, take account of the potential long-term impacts of short-term (and reactive) changes in the incentive structure faced by dentists (and, indeed, the public). Moreover, it appears that there has been a failure to accurately predict the *combined* impact of different policy changes.

But what does the evidence reveal about dental access and provision, and to what extent is it possible to attribute any changes to deliberate or unintended consequences of policy?

ACCESS TO NHS DENTISTRY

Access to NHS dental care will depend on a number of factors, and thus can be measured in a number of ways. Trends in four indicators – registrations (as an NHS patient), the supply of dentists, courses of treatment and private dental work – are examined below.

Registrations

The need to register with a dentist was introduced in October 1990. Until the last few years, the proportion of the population registered has remained fairly constant at about 50 per cent. Figure 1 shows trends in adult and child registrations since September 1992 for England and Wales. Child registrations have remained constant at 7.4 million (the 'saw-tooth' appearance of registrations is related to the movement of 16-year-olds into the category of adults at the end of each year).[1] In contrast, the number of adult registrations has declined progressively, falling from 23 million in 1993 to just over 18 million in March 1999 (a take-up rate of 46 per cent).

Changes in the length of the registration period (originally set at 24 months) have clearly had an impact on the total numbers registered. For example, the sharp decrease in adult registrations between December 1997 and October 1998 coincides with the completion of a changeover in the length of the registration period from 24 to 15 months. Increases in the number of adult 'lapses' (i.e. failures to re-register) also coincide with the registration changeover period. In addition to changes in the registration period, it has been suggested that recent decreases are also partly explained by better information.[2]

FIGURE 1

DENTAL REGISTRATIONS AND LAPSES IN REGISTRATIONS: ADULTS AND CHILDREN (ENGLAND AND WALES)

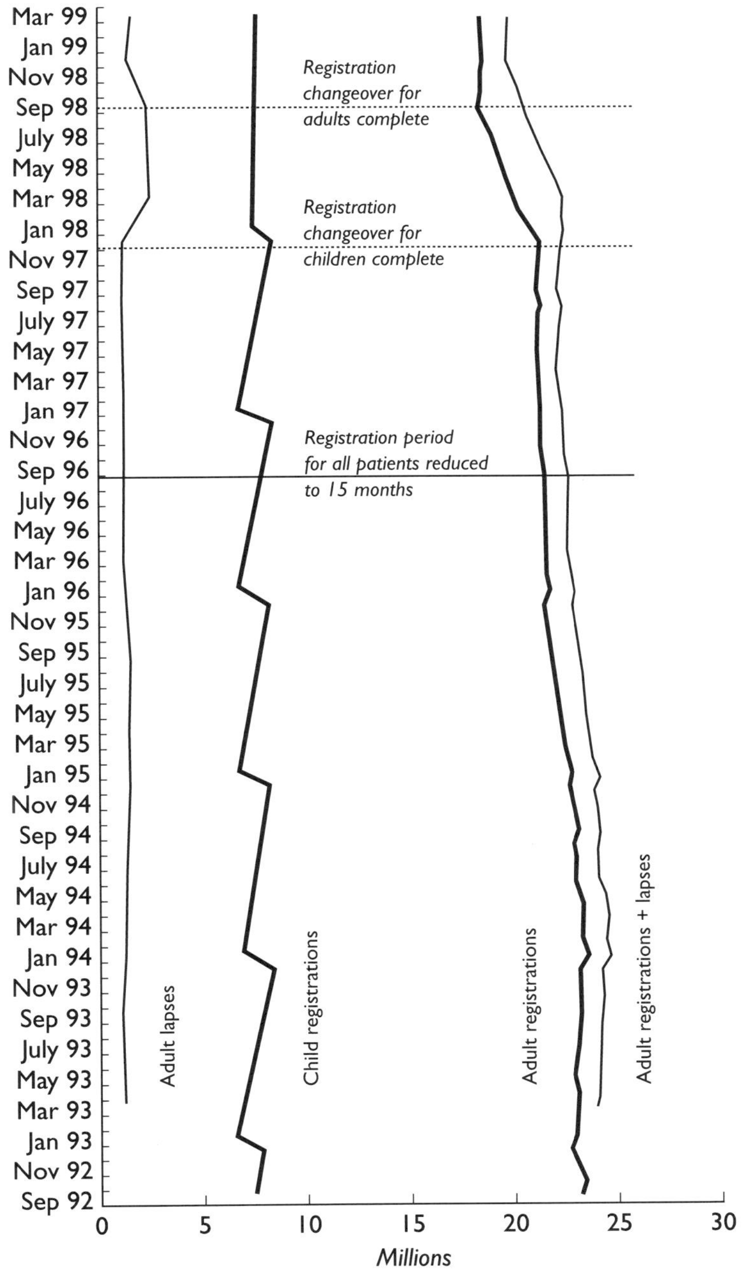

Since 1992, adult registrations have fallen by nearly 5 million – or over 20 per cent. Although changes in the registration period have been problematic for patients (many are unaware that their registration has lapsed[3]) and have exacerbated the problem of lapses, there is a clear long-term decline in the number of adults registered with a dentist as an NHS patient.

Part of the explanation for the decline in registrations is the apparent unwillingness of dentists to take people on as NHS patients. In a 1998 survey by the National Consumer Council, people across the country reported difficulty in finding a dentist who would register them for NHS care.[3] Just under one-fifth of those surveyed had tried to register with an NHS dentist in the previous year and, of these, one-third said they had experienced difficulty. Those with children under the age of 15 were more likely to have tried to find an NHS dentist (and to have had difficulty) than those without children. Geographical differences also emerged from the survey. In the south of England a quarter of those surveyed had tried to find an NHS dentist and 43 per cent of these said they had experienced problems. Class differences were also evident: those in lower socio-economic groups were more likely to have had difficulty than others.

Furthermore, a British Dental Association (BDA) survey of health authorities in England and Wales in 1998 found that about half of those responding reported an increase in the number of telephone calls from the public about problems finding a dentist, and half thought there was a local shortage of dentists.[4]

Numbers of dentists

Dental practitioners are legitimately registered as NHS dentists if they see only a few NHS patients or if they see children on the NHS but offer private treatment to adults. The number of dentists working within the general dental services has been steadily increasing. Between 1993 and 1998, the number of dentists in England and Wales increased by 500, from 15,800 to 16,300.[2] However these are not whole-time-equivalent figures (for which information is not available). The BDA believes that there is a shortage of dentists working in all branches of the NHS due to trends towards more part-time work.[5] The total number of NHS dentists therefore does not indicate the true size of the workforce providing NHS general dental services. By international comparisons, the number of dentists per head of population in the UK has been and remains relatively low (see Figure 2).

Courses of treatment

The number of adult courses of dental treatment per year has steadily increased over the last ten years, from 22.4 million in England and Wales in 1987 to 25.3 million in 1997, and has been cited as evidence to suggest there is not an access problem.[6] Table 1 shows these annual figures alongside the number of adult registrations for September each year and the average gross unit cost of adult treatments. As the number of treatments provided within the NHS increases, the unit cost falls, with an overall fall of 18 per cent over the ten-year period from 1987/88 to 1997/98. NHS dentists may well have to perform more procedures in order to maintain their income from item of service fees. Alternatively, the fall in unit cost could indicate more efficient delivery of care. However, the number of courses of treatment on its own is a poor indicator of access to services, as it does not show the number of individuals receiving care, or whether care was appropriate or even necessary.

FIGURE 2

DENTISTS PER 10,000 POPULATION: OECD COUNTRIES (1994)

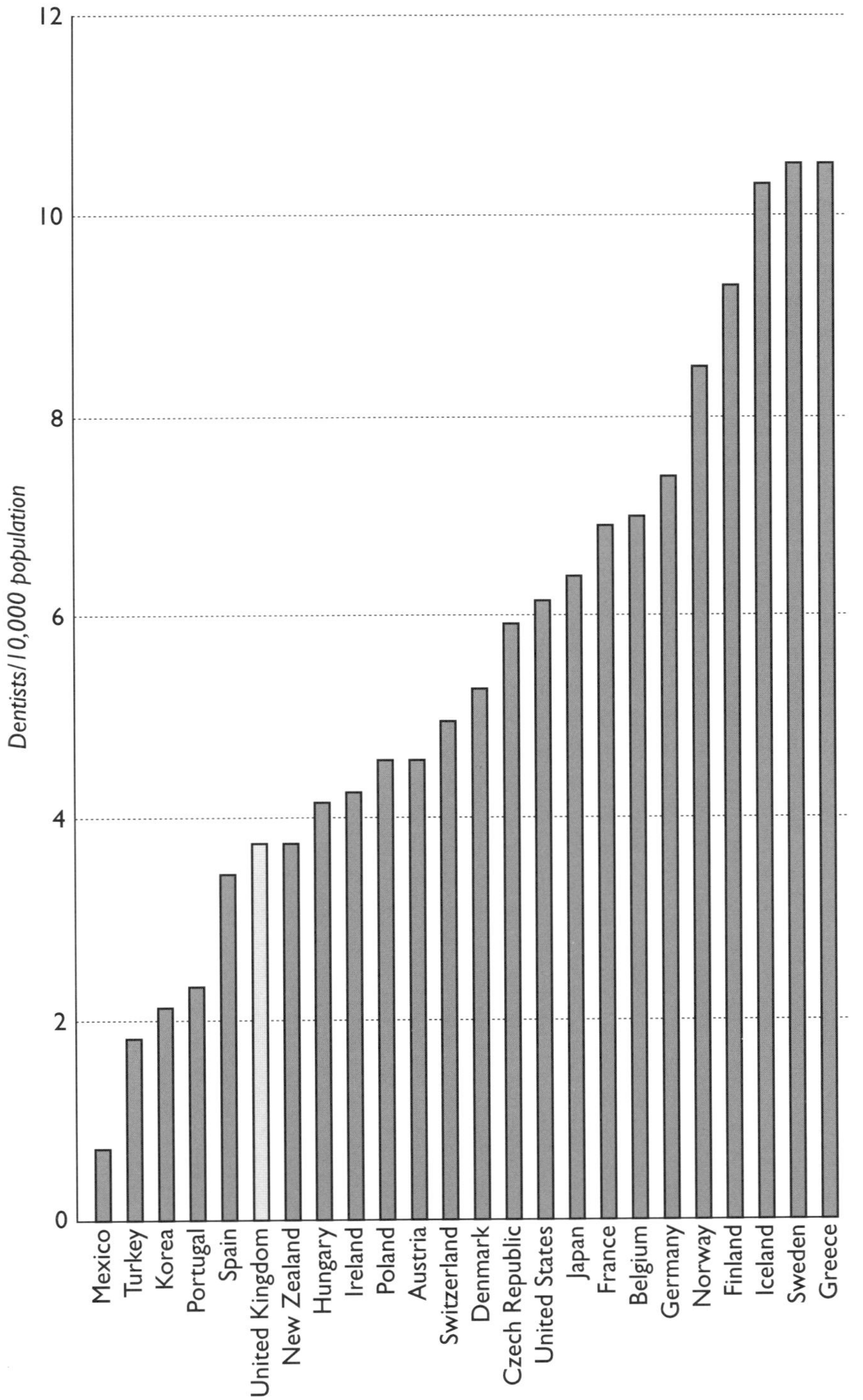

TABLE 1

KEY STATISTICS ON GENERAL DENTAL SERVICES

General dental services[1]	*1987–88*	*1993–94*	*1994–95*	*1995–96*	*1996–97*	*1997–98*	*% change 1987–88 to 1997–98*
Number of general dental practitioners[2] (30 September)	14,765	15,773	15,885	15,951	16,336	16,728	13
Adult courses of treatment (thousands)	22,395	24,848	24,913	24,752	24,580	25,268	13
Adults registered into continuing care (thousands) at 30 September[3]	n/a	21,530	21,050	19,994	19,524	19,383	n/a
Average gross cost of all adult courses of treatment (1997–98 prices) (£)	45	40	41	40	39	37	-18

Notes

1. General dental services are the care and treatment provided by independent high street dentists who provide services under arrangements made with health authorities.
2. Principals, assistants and vocational trainees.
3. Registrations only began with the introduction of the new dental contract from 1 October 1990. From September 1996, new registrations have a 15-month period, affecting registration numbers from December 1997 onwards.

Source: Department of Health. The Government's Expenditure Plans 1999-2000. London, Department of Health, 1999.

Private dental work

There is no doubt that dentists are performing more private work than before. A survey of dentists in England in 1998 found that over half the respondents (55 per cent) said they had increased the number of patients treated privately over the previous ten years.[7] This survey also showed that most change was reported by dentists for whom private patients already made up more than half their list. Those for whom private treatment was a minor part of their work continued to make it so. The BDA's *Business Trends* survey for the same year also showed that dentists were treating fewer patients on the NHS and performing more private treatments – evidence which the BDA cited in its annual submission to the Doctors and Dentists Review Body (DDRB) to support their claim for an increase in dentists' pay.[5] The Department of Health confirms that in 1992/93 private work accounted for only about 5 per cent of total gross earnings before expenses for dentists working on their own. But over the combined years 1995/96 and 1996/97 this proportion had increased to 25 per cent.[8]

Overall, the evidence on access appears somewhat mixed: adult registrations are declining, but children's are constant; also, the number of dentists has increased, as has the number of courses of dental treatment. But surveys suggest that the public have found it increasingly difficult to find a dentist willing to take them as NHS patients. Moreover, there is evidence that the volume of dental work carried out privately has increased. Problems of access appear to be centred on adults and in particular areas of the country. Whilst recent changes in the registration period have contributed to a fall in adult registrations as individuals fail to re-register, there are a number of other changes which, taken together, go some way towards explaining access difficulties. Two issues in particular are important: a change in the nature of the NHS dental contract and revisions to the payment system for dentists carrying out work on the NHS.

CONTRACTS AND PAYMENTS

For more than 40 years, dentists have been paid predominantly by item of service, but in 1990 their contract with the NHS was extensively altered to reflect the growing need for preventive as opposed to restorative work. Personal lists were introduced and a fixed payment offered for the routine care of children registered with each dentist (even if no treatments were given). For adults a fee per item was still paid, together with a continuing care payment for each registered patient. Dentists were generally unhappy about the 1990 changes, with predictions of 'supervised neglect' of children and 'cream skimming' if only children with healthy mouths were registered.

The effects of the new incentives presented by the 1990 contract were not fully predicted by the Department of Health. In 1991/92 actual net general dental service (GDS) spending was 25 per cent higher than predicted, and in 1992/93 nearly 20 per cent more (see Figure 3). Individual dentists received an average of £12,500 more than their target income for 1991/92.[7,9] Following this 'overspend' the Government attempted a claw-back, and proposed changes to the fee scale to try to engineer a 20 per cent reduction in the income of dentists in 1992/93.[9] In the event, the full claw-back was not implemented, and the dental fee scale was reduced by only 7 per cent. Nevertheless, the repercussions included widespread and vocal dissatisfaction within the dental profession. Members of the BDA voted to stop registering new NHS patients and to not accept charge-paying adults.[7] The miscalculation of their predicted pay (and the attempt to recover money by reducing fees) has had serious effects on dentists' sense of commitment to the NHS, with many feeling that they were penalised for working productively under their new contract.[7, 10]

FIGURE 3

GENERAL DENTAL SERVICE SPENDING: DIFFERENCE BETWEEN ESTIMATES AND OUTTURNS: GROSS AND NET (EXCLUDING PATIENT CHARGES)

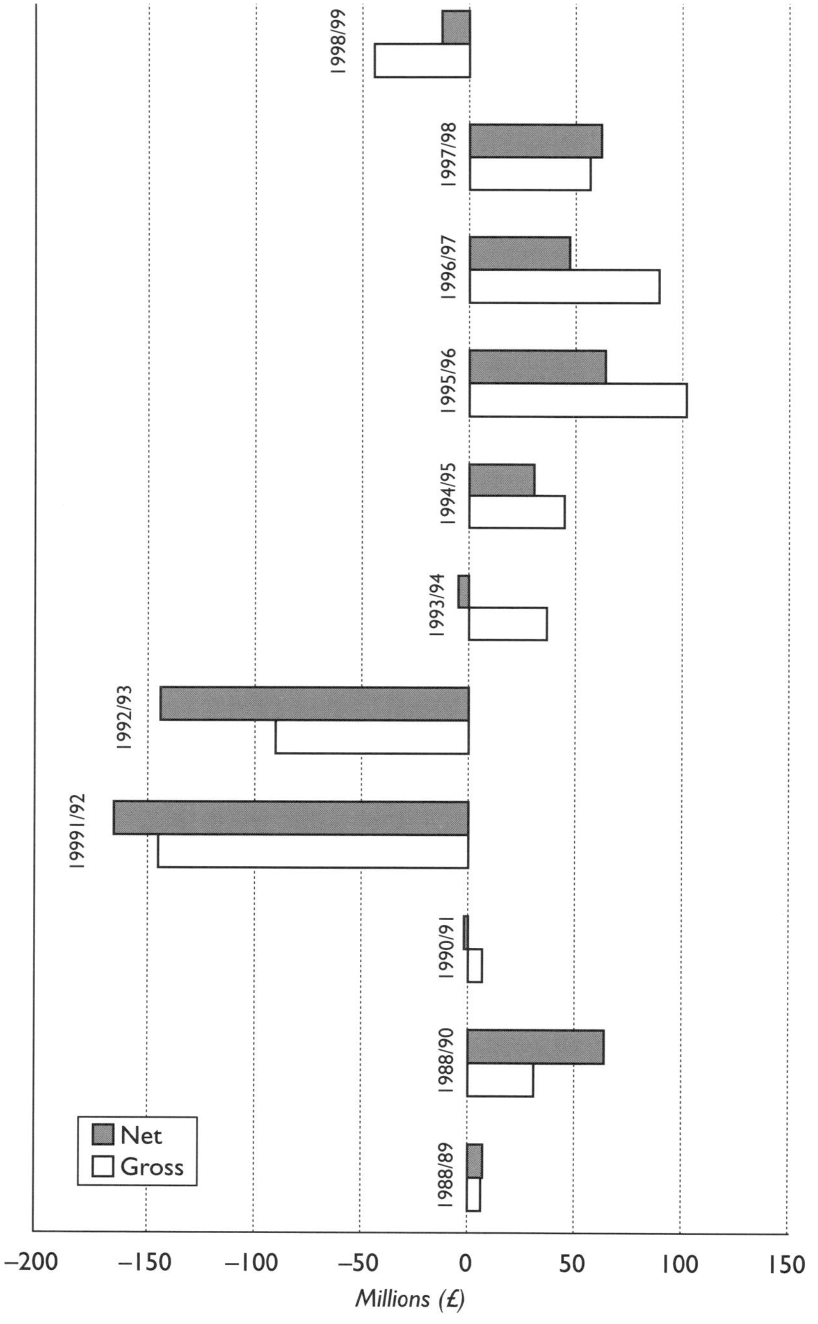

In 1994 the 'target income' approach (whereby the Department of Health set an average income for dentists based on a combination of fee scales and volume of work) was abandoned, and dentists' remuneration has since been determined solely by alterations to the scale of fees for items of work (recommendations for which are made by the DDRB each year). In 1996 there were further changes to the dentists' contract to soften the 1990 changes, notably a partial move back to a fee per item scale for children.

Despite the Government's attempts to improve the contract, the difficulties in the early 1990s appear to have encouraged dentists to question their commitment to the NHS and to look to alternative sources of income through the private sector.

Is there evidence that NHS dentists are no longer providing the volume of care that they used to? The number of adult NHS treatments has actually steadily increased over the last five years (see Table 1). However, this could mean that dentists are having to perform more NHS treatments per person registered in order to maximise NHS income, whilst still offering an increasing proportion of private care. A different (and indirect) indication of the volume of NHS dental care being provided each year can be obtained by looking at the financial performance of dentists in relation to their contract.

Following the large mismatch between predicted and actual GDS spending in 1991/92 and 1992/93, there followed five years in which the Department consistently overestimated total GDS spending (see Figure 3). It would appear that dentists as a group have, in some sense, under-performed in these years – that is, the volume of care they have provided has been less than expected. Disentangling the reasons for this is complicated by the number of factors that lie behind the GDS spending figures. For example, the 'underspends' may be a result of miscalculations by the Department, or real changes in the volume of work, changes in fee scales, or reductions in the number of dentists performing NHS work – or, more likely, a combination of all these factors.

STEPS TO IMPROVE ACCESS TO NHS DENTISTRY

Since 1993, various attempts have been made to tackle the problems generated by the new dental contract, the changes in dentists' remuneration and the issue of access to NHS dental care. In 1993 the Government commissioned a *Fundamental Review* by Sir Kenneth Bloomfield.[11] This was followed by a Health Select Committee report,[12] a White Paper in 1994 (*Improving NHS Dentistry*)[13] and a Departmental oral health strategy[14] in the same year. More recently, the new Labour Government initiated the *Investing in Dentistry*[15] strategy, in an attempt to boost flagging registrations in specific areas of the country.

Investing in Dentistry made money available over two years for health authorities to invest in grants towards dental practice expansion, improved facilities and equipment, start-up packages for newly trained dentists and for salaried options. In the event the grant approval process (in which dentists applied to health authorities, which in turn applied to the Department of Health) proved slow. In the first six months of the initiative (September 1997 to March 1998), of the £9 million available in that year only £3.8m had been approved, and a mere £175,000 actually paid out.[16] A total of £10 million was allocated for 1998/99, whereupon the scheme was curtailed. Overall, 279 funding requests were approved, and a total of £8.1 million in direct incentive payments was authorised with the objective of enabling 650,000 patients to register for NHS dental care.[17] Given the size of the de-registration problem – with 2 million fewer adults registered in early 1999 compared with 1997 – it is difficult to see how *Investing in Dentistry* could yet be judged a success.

A further initiative in 1997 – personal dental services (PDS) schemes – was introduced by the Government, whereby funding was offered to new primary care and specialist services in a number of pilot sites, using a local contract framework. The number of patients involved in the schemes so far is not large (less than 200,000) and it is too early to know if access will be enhanced.

Yet another attempt to deal with the problems that have beset NHS dentistry is promised by the Government before the end of 1999, with the publication of a new dental health strategy. It remains to be seen whether it will involve further financial incentives or contract changes to attract dentists back into the NHS and whether it will be informed by dental health need. The national Adult Dental Health Survey (carried out in 1998 and yet to be published) should capture important changes to dental public health that have taken place since the last survey in 1988.[18]

THE FUTURE

When the NHS first opened for business the two greatest demands were for dental care and spectacles. Ironically, these are two services that have progressively shifted out of the preserve of the NHS. Explanations for these shifts can be found in the policies of successive governments over the last ten to twenty years, which have set the economic environment for NHS dentistry. Informing these policies has been a combination of changes in the epidemiology of dental health and in dental technologies, which have begun to impact on dental health and change the nature of the profession itself.

A key high-level question for the Government's dental strategy to address, therefore, is the extent to which dentistry is allowed to drift further out of the orbit of the NHS, or whether coherent and workable attempts are made to secure equitable and universal access. Given the fundamental nature of these issues, public involvement in these decisions is essential. Unfortunately, the UK has a long tradition of avoiding such debates: deciding what is in and what is out of the NHS is, at one level, clearly difficult, but, as with rationing issues in other areas of the service, explicitness is preferable to implicitness.

REFERENCES

1. Dental Practice Board. *Registrations: GDS Quarterly Statistics*. Eastbourne: March, 1999.

2. Dental Practice Board. *Working Together: Annual Review 1997–98*. Eastbourne: Dental Practice Board, 1998.

3. National Consumer Council. *Consumer Concerns 1998. A consumer view of health services, the report of an RSL survey*. London: National Consumer Council, 1998.

4. British Dental Association. *Access to dental services and recruitment of salaried GDPs – a survey of health authorities*. London: British Dental Association, 1999.

5. British Dental Association. *Evidence to the Review Body on Doctors' and Dentists' Remuneration*. London: British Dental Association, 1998.

6. Department of Health. *The Government's Expenditure Plans 1999–2000*. London: The Stationery Office, 1999.

7. Silvester S, Calnan M, Manley G, Taylor-Gooby P. *Public or private? Practitioners' beliefs, values and practices*. Canterbury: Centre for Health Services Studies, University of Kent, December 1998.

8. Personal communication. London: Department of Health, June 1999.

9. Perri. *Open Wide: Futures for dentistry in 2010*. London: Demos, 1996.

10. Jackman J. Filling in. *Health Service Journal* 31 August 1995.

11. Sir Kenneth Bloomfield. *Fundamental Review of Dental Remuneration*. London: Department of Health, December 1992.

12. House of Commons health committee fourth report. *Dental Services*. London: HMSO, May 1993.

13. Department of Health. *Improving NHS Dentistry*. London: HMSO, 1994.

14. Department of Health. *An oral health strategy for England*. London: Department of Health, 1994.

15. NHS Executive. *Investing in Dentistry*. (HSG (97) 38). Leeds: NHS Executive, September 1997.

16. Denham M. Parliamentary answer to Jackie Ballard MP, 29 April 1999.

17. Denham M. Parliamentary answer to Jackie Ballard MP, 31 March 1999.

18. Todd JE, Lader D. *Adult dental health 1988: United Kingdom*. London: HMSO, 1991.

Personal Medical Services pilots: progress and prospects

A review of the first wave of PMS pilots, and a look at what the future holds for primary care institutions.

Clare Jenkins

As noted in last year's Health Policy Review, personal medical services (PMS) pilots were introduced in April 1998, following the passing of the NHS (Primary Care) Act 1997 just before the Labour Government came to power. The Act can be seen as a response to a widely held perception that the existing regime for primary care was too restrictive.

Despite, or perhaps because of, the imposition of the 1990 'New Contract' and the introduction of fundholding in the early 1990s, dissatisfaction with the structure and organisation of primary care services was widely expressed by health care professionals, managers and policy-makers.

The original GP national contract (known as the 'Red Book'), much of which had been in place since 1948, was increasingly seen as a strait-jacket, preventing innovation and development in primary care. More flexibility was called for to provide services that would meet specific local needs, particularly in deprived areas such as the inner city. There were also widespread calls for rigid employment framework for GPs to be overhauled.

The publication of *Primary Care – the future* followed a listening exercise carried out by the Conservative Government early in 1996. In October of that year, after an agenda-setting round of seminars, the White Paper *Choice and Opportunity* was published. The 1997 Act provided the called-for flexibilities on a selective basis.

HOW MANY PMS PILOTS ARE THERE?

The Department of Health received 567 expressions of interest from projects keen to use the flexibilities offered by the new Act.[1] Of these, 123 full applications were subsequently submitted.[2] That less than a quarter of those projects originally expressing an interest went forward to submit a formal proposal was largely due to the fact that many of the projects simply did not require the new Act's provisions. For other prospective pilots, concerns were voiced over the right of return to GMS and the impact of PMS on pensions – issues that were slow to be resolved. The popular press printed negative comments and there was opposition from sections of the medical profession towards the pilots. The timing of the PMS initiative meant that it was overshadowed by the introduction of the Labour Government's new health policy: the pilots were launched into a Health Service focused on the setting up of primary care groups (PCGs), and some potential pilots decided to 'wait and see' before committing themselves.

One hundred personal medical services (PMS) pilots were given the go-ahead by the Secretary of State to 'go live' in April 1998. Of these, 17 pilots decided not to proceed with their projects, for a variety of reasons.[1] Some pilots had found it difficult to finalise local contracts and launch complex projects in the short timescales given (there were only 11 months between submitting an expression of interest and 'going live'[3]). Other pilots reported disagreements with their health authority over funding or over the existence of the pilot altogether. In other cases, the pilots experienced difficulty in appointing suitable GP candidates. One pilot withdrew from the scheme after a year because the rationale behind their project had been overtaken by the development of their local PCG. Of the original expressions of interest, therefore, less than one in five were given permission to go live, and of this 'successful' 100 almost 20 per cent were not in operation at the end of the first 12 months.

WHERE ARE THEY?

The PMS pilots are not located evenly across the country. Over half of the 82 English PMS pilots remaining in operation in year two are in the north and the Midlands, while the majority of those in the south and west of the country are to be found in the London region. As a policy, PMS was introduced to raise standards in under-served areas, and to increase accessibility to primary care services. Initial analysis showed that PMS pilots appeared to be providing primary care services in areas where deprivation levels are higher than the English average, and this was particularly true for the nurse-led and community trust-managed pilots.[4]

EXAMPLES OF PMS PILOTS

PMS pilots have taken a number of organisational forms. The following examples from London illustrate how varied the first-wave pilots were.

In Lambeth, an inner city area of south London, a new practice was set up by a community trust to provide services for refugees, asylum seekers, the homeless and drug users living in hostels in the area. Such marginalised populations are likely to experience difficulty in accessing traditional GMS services. When visiting the new practice, patients are routinely seen by a nurse practitioner, who assesses whether they need referring on to one of the practice's two GPs.

In a more affluent part of south west London, seven practices, with 39 partners, formed a merged partnership 'super practice' to provide 'PMS-plus' services to their patients. The practices planned to build on achievements they made as a total purchasing pilot (TPP), using the flexibilities offered by PMS to appoint a pharmaceutical adviser and mental health facilitator. They also hoped to increase their use of intermediate care facilities, develop an integrated nursing team, introduce personal development plans for staff and streamline their administrative structures.

The PMS pilots that 'went live' in April 1998 were able to take advantage of a range of new ways of working:

Local contracts

PMS pilots negotiate their own contracts locally with their health authority. The contracts may be one of two types: 'PMS' practices provide the same broad range of services as traditional GMS practices; 'PMS-plus' practices can extend their contract to include a range of other services, for example community nursing. PMS pilot funding is drawn from the national GP pool (using the pilots' historical income, where appropriate, as an initial guide), and is cash-limited at the health authority level.

Salaried doctors

GPs in the UK have fiercely guarded their status as self-employed 'independent contractors'. Over recent years, calls for a salaried option have increased, particularly among younger GPs for whom the financial and managerial responsibility of owning, or renting, surgery premises and employing their own staff may be unattractive. PMS introduces the option for GPs to be employed on a salaried basis. However, except in specific circumstances, if the PMS salaried option is chosen, all GPs in a practice must take on

PMS status – it is not an opportunity to mix GMS and PMS within a practice.

NEW PROVIDERS

The introduction of PMS pilots allowed a range of new providers to enter the primary care arena. Ten of the original 100 PMS pilots were nurse-led or nurse-partnership projects where nurses had the opportunity to run their own practices and employ GPs. Around a third of the pilots were managed by trusts, both community and acute. In addition, the 1997 Act allowed private companies to propose pilots, and BUPA, Unichem and Healthcall were amongst a number of organisations reported to have expressed interest. However, this option was later withdrawn and all projects had to be proposed by members of the 'NHS family'.

WHAT DOES THE FUTURE HOLD FOR PMS PILOTS?

PMS pilots are due to run for three years before any decision is made concerning their long-term future. One of the stipulations the Government made when the sites were launched was that learning emerging from the PMS initiative was to be reviewed through local and national evaluations.[5] Local evaluations carried out by the sites themselves, sometimes in partnership with other research organisations, are likely to be small-scale and experimental in nature. The national evaluation, on the other hand, is centrally funded, and involves four separate projects co-ordinated by the National Primary Care Research and Development Centre (NPCRDC).[5] The national projects aim to address strategic policy issues by considering the characteristics and experiences of the pilots, and involving all the PMS sites.

PMS pilots have been 'live' for just over a year and, although early learning has started to emerge,[6] it is too early to say how successful they have been.

PMS pilots were originally a policy of the previous Government and have, at times, appeared to slip down the current administration's political agenda. The future of a possible second wave was uncertain and, when announced, the start-date was put back by six months to allow a clear run for PCGs to establish themselves. The PMS pilot initiative now appears to be favoured by the Government, and is seen as an important test-ground for learning to be passed on to PCGs and primary care trusts (PCTs).[7] The Secretary of State has particularly called for second-wave pilot proposals from salaried initiatives and new forms of practice-based contracts offering other professionals, particularly nurses, the 'opportunity to be full partners and explore the better use of skill mix'.[7] The successful second-wave applications are due to be announced at the end of June and will 'go live' in October 1999. It will be interesting to see how the new pilot projects will build on the innovations and experiences of the 100 first-wave pioneers.

REFERENCES

1. Department of Health press release 1997/151. Alan Milburn announces Primary Care Act pilots. 1 July 1997.

2. Personal communication. Leeds: NHSE, 11 November 1998.

3. Department of Health. *Personal Medical Services pilots under the NHS (Primary Care) Act 1997. A comprehensive guide*. NHSE, 1997.

4. Lewis R, Gillam S, editors. *Transforming Primary Care: Personal Medical Services and the new NHS*. London: King's Fund, 1999.

5. Department of Health. *Personal Medical Services pilots under the NHS (Primary Care) Act 1997, a guide to local evaluation*. NHSE, 1997.

6. Lewis R, Jenkins C, Gillam S. *Personal Medical Services pilots: rewriting the Red Book*. London: King's Fund, 1999.

7. Department of Health. *Personal Medical Services pilots under the NHS (Primary Care) Act 1997. A comprehensive guide*. Second edition. NHSE, 1998.

NHS networks: rational technology or Triffid?

Information for Health promised much but implementation has been slow and the outcome may be very different to the centralised approach originally envisaged.

Justin Keen

For people interested in NHS information systems, 1998 was dominated by the publication of a new information strategy, Information for Health.1 It was trailed for most of the year, before being published in September, when much of the initial comment about it was positive. Some of the news was undoubtedly welcome: there was some money for implementation and the previous focus on administrative data was to be shifted to clinical data. Yet, by the middle of 1999, things seemed to have gone flat, and it was apparent that we were still waiting for key strategic decisions. Familiar-sounding stories of problems were also emerging – particularly over one of the flagship initiatives, the dedicated NHS network, NHSnet. This article examines the developing story of NHSnet, which exemplifies the tension between the central desire to implement systems quickly and the continuing difficulties of implementation in the NHS.

THE NEW STRATEGY

On first encounter, the vision of a dedicated network for the distribution of data within the NHS seems sensible. If you have a single network that everyone can use, then all users know what systems they need to link to the network and, once linked, can talk to everyone else. *Information for Health* states that:

> *... the development of the NHS 'Information Superhighway' is a major deliverable in The New NHS. The NHSnet has the potential to deliver the enormous benefits of information technology to all parts of the NHS ... A private managed service offers the potential of a faster and much more consistent and reliable service [than the Internet].* (p.53)

In fact this part of the strategy is not really new – the PFI contracts for NHS-wide networking were signed with BT Syntegra and other firms in 1995. Until this year the use of most of the network was charged for, but there were concerns about data security; NHS sites had found the charges too high – it could be cheaper to use a dispatch bike to send a data tape from a trust to a health authority; and there had been considerable resistance to using it. The NHS Executive has now agreed to pay all of the charges centrally, partly in order to achieve one of its key objectives – connecting to all general practices by the end of 1999.

The NHS Executive has also published a number of guidance documents in recent months on such matters as connecting GPs to NHSnet[2] and information systems requirements for primary care groups.[3] Most of the money earmarked for information systems in the Modernisation Fund (£40 million out of £50 million) is for primary care.[4] Overall, these documents are being used to paint a favourable picture of the value of NHSnet and, particularly, its role in connecting general practices into a national network.

PROBLEMS

The positive vision sits uneasily with the emerging evidence. The NHS Executive announced in March 1999 that there was to be a 'performance review' of NHSnet in the light of published reports of operational difficulties. The National Audit Office (NAO) reported that less than 10 per cent of general practices were connected to NHSnet in April 1999[5] and the NHS in Northern Ireland has decided to abandon the use of NHSnet, on the basis that it is too expensive (in spite of the removal of usage charges).[6] Comments made to the author by users suggest that: it is still too slow and unreliable to support clinical work, comparing unfavourably with the Internet in some eyes (which is not perfect either); it is expensive for GPs to link to it, because the 'hidden' costs within practices are high; and there are continuing concerns in the field about data security and confidentiality. Given that the contracts for NHSnet have been in place for almost four years, this situation must give cause for concern.

The National Audit Office Report

There is a deeper, and in many ways more interesting, story behind the current concerns. The NAO Report on the 1992 and 1998 IM&T strategies noted that the only full business case is for electronic patient records. Other components of the strategy do not have full business cases, and there is not a full business case for the strategy as a whole. The latter point is critical, because the overall case would provide the economic rationale for the particular combination of technologies the NHS is being told to implement. The Treasury has allowed the strategy to go ahead on the condition that the NHS Executive prepares individual project business cases on the components of the strategy (and on the strategy as a whole) and undertakes proper evaluations of them. But these cannot realistically be done in time to influence implementation, if the tight timetables in *Information for Health* are to be achieved.

On the NHS-wide networking strategy, the NAO further noted that the business case objectives:

> *...do not make clear what the project is expected to achieve and do not provide anything against which progress can be judged.* (p.60)

So, NHSnet has been allowed to continue without any clear sense of what it is supposed to do, or any built-in criteria for judging its success. The value of the PFI contracts has not been published, but the NAO records £26.8 million expenditure in the period to March 1998 (i.e. over some 30 months), which suggests that the contracts are worth some £65–£70 million over seven years. There must be a risk that the NHS is implementing major systems with high costs and few benefits; business cases do not guarantee to avoid this, but ought to reduce the probability of bad investments.

This story is unfolding against a backdrop of well-documented problems with NHS information and communications technologies (ICTs) in the past decade,[7, 8] and research evidence that ICTs do not yield substantial benefits in health care settings.[9, 10] There is, then, a clear clash between a set of favourable beliefs about ICTs and the awkward realities of the NHS. This tends to confirm arguments made in *Health Care UK* last year that believers in ICTs view them as a special case, which is deemed not to need the usual paraphernalia of business cases and formal approvals:[11] they are going to be implemented, and that is that. Strong supporters of ICTs, including the Prime Minister,[12] continue with their support in spite of serious technical problems with current and past systems, and evidence that costs outweigh benefits in major projects.

'THE DAY OF THE TRIFFIDS'?

It may be fruitful to think about NHSnet as a contest between different types of rationality. On the one hand there is a top-down vision, underpinned by an unshakeable belief in the value of ICTs, where the only problem is those awkward GPs who keep objecting to the NHS Executive's sensible plans. On the other had there is a more bottom-up and organic vision. Here, ICTs are like slow-growing ivy, which over time grow to cover the whole of the NHS. However the centre sees such developments to be more like Triffids, which threaten the whole fabric and which must therefore be controlled as tightly as possible. The real clash, on this view, is between the way we do things now and the way we will do things when the Triffids are all around us. ICTs bring with them a change in the way that organisations work, something that many people find uncomfortable, but will get used to in the end. The central vision does not take account of this clash – even though it is obvious to those in the NHS.

For an academic commentator this is familiar territory: such classic works as Burns and Stalker[13] highlight the co-existence of formal organisational processes with more informal, contingent ones. ICTs look like they are part of the rational, formal world, but are really part of the messy and contingent one. This creates real problems for those at the centre, both in terms of managing implementation and in measuring costs and benefits. Management can only really succeed if it is local, and go at a pace that fits in with other demands on management and clinical time – which *Information for Health* recognises in places, but does not act on, preferring instead to set a demanding implementation timetable.

CONCLUDING COMMENT

NHSnet embodies the tension between a rational central vision of ICTs and a messy reality. It is difficult to argue with positions that are grounded in a strong ideology, but it does now seem imperative that supporters of ICTs take a serious look at the costs of their preferred technologies. Northern Ireland's decision to withdraw from NHSnet, in spite of the removal of tolls, stresses the point that the 'hidden' costs of implementation within general practices are high, and currently perceived to be too high a price to pay for the benefits of joining. For the centre, the logic of its own position is that ICTs are worth having, and so should be paid for somehow – if GPs will not pay, then the centre should be happy to pay for them. To some extent it is doing this, but Northern Ireland is saying that the sums are not enough.

In the absence of major additional investments in this area, the likelihood now is that local sites will continue to develop their own solutions, much as some have been doing since the mid-1990s, when they decided to stop waiting for decisions and money for the 1992 strategy. A number of groups of general practices already have their own links to local hospitals, some PCGs already have their own intranets, and there are *ad hoc* developments in areas such as telemedicine that may be the precursors of widely-used systems in the future. Sites are putting in systems driven by local needs and their judgements about what is worth doing. Put another way, there may well be an economic logic in developing outwards from local networks. It might be slow and messy in places, but the NHS will get there in the end – and in all probability at around the ten-year mark originally set by the centre.

REFERENCES

1. NHS Executive. *Information for Health*. London: NHS Executive, 1998.

2. NHS Executive. *Information Management and Technology Requirements to Support Primary Care Groups*. Leeds: NHS Executive, 1999.

3. NHS Executive. *Implementing Information for Health. Connecting General Practices to NHSnet; Resources for Health Informatics Services*. Health Service Circular 1999/094. Leeds: NHSE, 1999.

4. *Modern Public Services for Britain: Investing in Reform. Comprehensive Spending Review: New Public Spending Plans 1999–2002*. Cmnd 4011. London: HMSO, 1998.

5. National Audit Office. *The 1992 and 1998 Information Management and Technology Strategies*

of the NHS Executive. London: Stationery Office, 1999.

6. Dunne R. Ulster scraps NHSnet plans due to cost. *Doctor* 11 June 1999: 2.

7. National Audit Office. *Department of Health: The Hospital Information Support Systems Initiative*. London: HMSO, 1996.

8. National Audit Office. *NHS Executive: The Purchase of the Read Codes and the Management of the NHS Centre for Coding and Classification*. London: Stationery Office, 1998.

9. Sullivan F, Mitchell E. Has general practitioner computing made a difference to patient care? A systematic review of published reports. *BMJ* 1995; 311: 848–52.

10. Hunt DL, Haynes RB, Hanna SE, Smith K. Effects of computer-based clinical decision support systems on physician performance and patient outcomes: a systematic review. *JAMA* 1998; 280: 1339–46.

11. Keen J. Should the NHS have a computing strategy? In: Harrison A, editor. *Health Care UK 1997/98*. London: King's Fund, 1998: 164–77.

12. Prime Minister. Modernising Public Services. Speech by the Prime Minister on 26 January 1999. Available at the 10 Downing Street Internet site (www.number-10.gov.uk).

13. Burns T, Stalker G. *The Management of Innovation*. Oxford: Oxford University Press, 1994.

Self-regulation of health professionals: the need for a coherent framework

The individual professions retain their own regulatory structures: a uniform approach is required.

Juan I Baeza

Ever since the General Medical Council's (GMC) hearings on the Bristol case, a day has hardly gone by without a story of a 'dangerous doctor' or an incompetent nurse or physiotherapist in the daily papers. The public is being presented with daily reminders that their doctor or nurse could actually be damaging their health rather than being the trustworthy professional who can relieve pain and suffering. This damning media portrayal of a few poorly performing individuals damages the reputations of the vast majority of health professionals, who provide their patients with the highest level of care and treatment. However, this situation is more the fault of the Government, the individual professions and their professional regulatory bodies than an unfair and vindictive press. It has been the regulatory bodies' apparent inertia, lack of transparency and ineffectiveness in the field of managing poor performance that has in general led to the media vilification of heath professionals.

The Health Act 1999 grants the Secretary of State for Health broad order-making powers that may be used to reform the regulatory system for health professionals. These powers will allow him/her to more easily amend certain functions and structures of the professional health regulatory bodies. This should be welcomed as it allows the Secretary of State to adjust the roles of the various regulatory bodies more quickly, rather than having to make parliamentary time for primary legislation, which has taken many years in the past. Many of the changes that are suggested here could be carried out using this order-making power, although it should be used only after proper public and professional consultation.

Up to now, professional self-regulation within the health care sector has been seen as the concern of each profession in isolation from the others. This paper argues that the functions and procedures of bodies such as the GMC, the UK Central Council for Nurses, Midwives and Health Visitors (UKCC), the Council for Professions Supplementary to Medicine (CPSM) and others need to be examined in a coherent way. There should be a regulatory framework for health care as a whole as opposed to the various different and unco-ordinated regulatory mechanisms for each profession. This article argues that the functions of such a framework should be informed by a clear view of the purpose of professional self-regulation, which will help develop a set of principles that will address the current problems of professional self-regulation within the health care sector.

THE PURPOSE OF SELF-REGULATION

When self-regulation within the medical profession began in 1858 with the Medical Registration Act, its primary aim was to protect doctors from competition from other nonregistered practitioners. However, professional self-regulation is now sanctioned by the state on the grounds that it is the best method of protecting the public. The state has given certain professions the privilege to regulate themselves. In return these professions set up systems to ensure their members display high standards of professional behaviour and censure those who fall below these standards. For many years it has seemed that the public has been satisfied, or at least has been unconcerned, with the mechanisms for the self-regulation of doctors and other health professionals. The Merrison Report, which the Government set up in 1975 to look into the self-regulation of the medical profession, described the public–professional relationship of the time as:

> ... *a contract between the public and the profession, by which the public go to the profession for medical treatment because the profession has made sure it will provide satisfactory treatment.*[1]

As we approach the millennium it seems that the public no longer has such a trusting view of the medical profession and other health professionals. This contract needs to be re-examined to take account of a changed public attitude towards the professions. Although the purpose of professional self-regulation has changed from safeguarding professional interests to safeguarding the public interest, the mechanisms in place are suited more to the former than the latter. It is this discrepancy that needs addressing.

Successive governments have failed to examine professional self-regulation in a comprehensive manner. In the absence of any rational approach to the system of self-regulation, changes have been disjointed and incremental. These changes have resulted in a patchwork of highly variable mechanisms across the different professions, inflexible rules, decisions that lack transparency and regulatory arrangements that promote public scepticism.

Many of the problems with medical self-regulation were identified over 25 years ago. In 1972 a small panel of doctors published a report that called for a reformed GMC.[2] These doctors argued that the GMC should establish procedures to enable the monitoring of doctors' continuing competence to practice. It has taken the GMC more than 25 years to establish such procedures, illustrating the slowness of necessary reforms.

The main stakeholders (the professions, the professional bodies, the Government and the public) are all agreed that the purpose of professional regulation should be the protection of the public. There is arguably less agreement on whether regulation should take the form of self-regulation or outside regulation. However, both the current Government and previous ones have made it clear that self-regulation is their preferred option.[3] The aim now, therefore, should be to identify the main deficiencies in the current structures and propose some possible remedies to produce a coherent system of self-regulation rather than the current regulatory muddle.

THE PROBLEMS THAT NEED ADDRESSING

The first deficiency in the current arrangements is that the various regulatory bodies have inconsistent structures and approaches. There seems little reason for this lack of consistency apart from historical accident. There is no evidence base for any of these structures or any knowledge regarding the most effective way of carrying out the different bodies' responsibilities. It would seem that past governments have been at fault in this area, as many of the regulatory bodies (the CPSM being a good example) have spent many years lobbying government for changes to their statutory responsibilities.[4]

There are large variations between the various health regulatory bodies in terms of numbers and types of members, their disciplinary mechanisms and their lines of accountability. There is no reason why the different structures and memberships should vary in the ways that they do since the aims of these bodies are very similar. A standard framework for all the regulatory bodies in terms of membership and accountability would address this problem of consistency. Variations should exist only when this would support the work of a particular body. A working party could be set up to look at experiences from other professional bodies and other countries in order to determine the mechanisms that work best. The Government's White Paper on the social services[5] states that it will establish a General Social Care Council that will set conduct and practice standards for all social services staff. There is no reason why a similar council could not be set up in the health care sector. The Government has expressed the need to minimise variations in health care provision. Variations in the regulation of the health care professions should also be minimised.

A second deficiency is that there is little co-ordination or communication amongst the different regulatory bodies. There should be a multidisciplinary regulatory system to reflect the fact that multidisciplinary teams are responsible for delivering modern health care. The lack of such a regulatory system makes if difficult to deal with poorly performing multidisciplinary teams. Again, something similar to the proposed General Social Care Council could be a way of spreading best practice across the various professions and could help establish some consistency in approach for all the health care professions. An umbrella structure for the professional regulatory bodies could be a way of co-ordinating the various regulatory mechanisms. The current absence of any links between the regulatory bodies and the NHS complaints, disciplinary and Ombudsman systems would also be remedied by such a structure. The umbrella body could also act as a filter for public complaints and be the common public face for the various regulatory bodies. Such a structure would be better equipped to admit new professional bodies or allow the existing bodies to take on the regulation of other professions. There is currently a call for the regulation of health care assistants; the coherent framework that is suggested here would be better able to respond constructively to such calls.

A third deficiency that needs to be tackled is the lack of transparency in the current regulatory bodies' procedures. Although disciplinary hearings are open to the public, the screening processes that take place before the hearings are shrouded in unnecessary secrecy. There are no explanations given to complainants whose complaints are dismissed at the screening stage, before a full disciplinary hearing takes place. This lack of openness in the current regulatory bodies' complaint processes gives outsiders the perception that the system is unfair and is there to protect professional interests rather than those of the public. The whole complaints system should be open to public scrutiny so as to give the public confidence in a system that is there to protect their interests.

A FRAMEWORK OF PROFESSIONAL SELF-REGULATION

We have argued that there should be a consistent regulatory framework covering all the professions responsible for the delivery of health services, and that the prime aim of its self-regulation is to protect the public. If this objective is to be achieved, and be achieved visibly – hence commanding public confidence – the framework itself should be based on the following principles:

1. The workings of the system should be transparent so that the reasons for the decisions that are taken by the regulatory bodies can be understood and be open to scrutiny
2. Fairness should be at the centre of a regulatory system: procedures should be fair to both the professionals concerned and the complainants
3. A system whose aim is to protect the public must command its confidence. One way of securing this is for the various bodies to have a substantial lay membership, which will be able to promote the public's views on discussions and procedures. The lay members

should not merely be non-health professionals; they should be the voice for the various sectors of society. To this end, they should include representatives from patient organisations, ethnic minorities, disability organisations and consumer groups
4. The framework should be flexible so the mechanisms are able to reflect future changes in health care and society
5. Evidence-based health care is becoming the hallmark of modern health care. There is no reason why modern regulatory systems should not also be influenced by evidence of best practice. This could come either from experiences from abroad or from other self-regulating professions
6. Finally, the systems that are established for professional self-regulation must be practical so that they can carry out the work that they have been set up to do and not become a bureaucratic mess.

Changes to the professional regulatory systems are overdue. The Government has started to take a lead in this process with the Professions Allied to Medicine (PAMs) and the nursing professions. It has responded to the two reports published by JM Consulting, which were commissioned to review the regulatory bodies that cover nurses and the PAMs.[6, 7] In the light of these reports, it proposes to abolish current legislation and accept the majority of the two reports' recommendations, which will form the basis of two new Acts. A single UK-wide body will replace the UKCC and the four National Nursing Boards, and new powers will be introduced to ensure fitness to practice. The CPSM will also be similarly reformed to allow it to better regulate the expanding number of different professions that fall under the PAMs heading.[4]

But these measures simply continue the profession-by-profession approach. The whole issue of self-regulation needs to be examined in a coherent and comprehensive way. The incremental and fragmented way in which different parts of the system have been looked at up to now has been found lacking. It is time for so-called 'joined-up-government' in this area of health policy. The current Government is keen to modernise the NHS; this modernisation process should include the organisational aspects of professional self-regulation. The two guiding aims of such a process should be to minimise variation in the mechanisms the various regulatory bodies employ and to strengthen the public protection functions of these bodies. Although the Government has started the process of change in this important area, their approach of piecemeal change is likely to address only certain deficiencies and risks leaving the system as a whole in its present state of confusion.

REFERENCES

1. Salter B. *The politics of change in the health service*. Hampshire: Macmillan Press, 1998.

2. Klein R. *Complaints Against Doctors: a study of professional accountability*. London: Charles Knight, 1973.

3. Department of Health. *The New NHS Modern, Dependable*. London: The Stationery Office, 1997.

4. Harris C. Toeing the line. *Health Service Journal* 1999; 319: 24–25.

5. Department of Health. *Modernising Social Services*. London: The Stationery Office, 1998.

6. JM Consulting. *The regulation of health professions: report of a review of the Professions Supplementary to Medicine Act (1960) with recommendations for new legislation*. Bristol: JM Consulting, 1996.

7. JM Consulting. *The Regulation of Nurses, Midwives and Health Visitors*. Bristol: JM Consulting, 1998.

NICE and CHI: reducing variations and raising standards

NICE and CHI are at the centre of the Government's drive to raise standards of care and rebuild public confidence in the NHS. The new organisations will have to overcome a number of problems to achieve these aims.

Angela Coulter

The plans outlined in the 1997 White Paper[1] to put quality at the heart of the National Health Service have been widely welcomed, but how easy will it be to put them into practice, and how likely is it that the Government's goals will be achieved? At the centre of the Government's drive to promote equitable access and raise quality standards in the NHS are two new bodies: the National Institute of Clinical Excellence (NICE) and the Commission for Health Improvement (CHI). It is intended that these bodies will be part of a 'policy sandwich', the outer layers of which place considerable emphasis on national standard setting and monitoring (through the national service frameworks, the national performance framework and the National Patient and User Survey). The main sandwich filling is provided by the new system of clinical governance, in which trusts and primary care groups are required to demonstrate that they have effective quality improvement procedures in place, but this is to be supplemented by stronger systems for professional self-regulation and lifelong learning (see Box 1).

BOX 1: SETTING, DELIVERING, MONITORING STANDARDS

National Institute for Clinical Excellence
National service frameworks

Professional self-regulation	Clinical governance	Lifelong learning

Commission for Health Improvement
National performance framework

Source: Secretary of State for Health. *The New NHS: modern, dependable*. London: The Stationery Office, 1997.

This article considers the tasks facing these new organisations and some of the problems they will have to overcome if they are to achieve the objectives that have been set for them.

THE GOVERNMENT'S AIMS

The aims of the new policies were set out in *The New NHS* White Paper:

- to reduce variations in access to treatment
- to develop and implement national quality standards
- to ensure that services are responsive to patients' needs and preferences
- to promote efficiency and value for money
- to make quality the driving force in decision-making
- to rebuild public confidence in the NHS.

This list encompasses each of the six dimensions of quality – effectiveness, acceptability, efficiency, access, equity and relevance – which command wide support as goals for the Health Service.[2] Statements from ministers have laid particular stress on the need to promote equity of access to particular treatments or services and to tackle poor standards of clinical care. Public concern has been fuelled by media coverage of 'postcode prescribing' and geographical inequities in the provision of particular treatments, and by scandals such as the poor results obtained by cardiac surgeons treating children in Bristol. These stories drew attention to variations in the decision-making procedures of local health authorities and the failure of professional self-regulation mechanisms to ensure uniformly high standards of clinical care. Secretary of State Frank Dobson called for an end to 'the unacceptable variations that have grown up in recent years'[3] and announced a new 'statutory duty of quality' under which trust boards were to be held accountable for the quality of clinical care in their institutions.

THE NATIONAL INSTITUTE FOR CLINICAL EXCELLENCE

NICE has been set up to provide guidance to the NHS on clinical effectiveness, cost-effectiveness and clinical audit methods. Its aim is to 'produce clear guidance for clinicians about which treatments work best for which patients.[3] It has three broad functions:

- to appraise new and existing health technologies
- to develop and disseminate clinical guidelines
- to oversee clinical audit and confidential inquiries.

It is envisaged that NICE will eventually produce a range of clinical guidance 'products', some of which will focus on the treatment of specific conditions, while others will provide guidance on new treatments or products, including pharmaceuticals, devices, diagnostic tests and surgical procedures.

In outlining his plans for the new institute, its Chairman, Sir Michael Rawlins, argued that the provision of a single, authoritative source of advice would mean that postcode prescribing 'should largely become a thing of the past'.[4] There are a number of reasons why this optimistic forecast may turn out to be difficult to achieve. The main problems NICE will have to overcome are the limited extent and nature of the evidence on which to base its judgements, and political difficulties caused by the Government's refusal to acknowledge the inevitability of rationing.

EVIDENCE PROBLEMS

The tasks for NICE were set out in some detail in a discussion paper produced by the NHS Executive entitled *Faster access to modern treatment*.[5] This outlined the need for timely guidance on individual treatments and products, to avoid:

- slow uptake of beneficial new treatments
- geographical variations in the use of treatments due to different interpretations of the evidence on clinical and cost-effectiveness
- wasteful use of treatments that are not clinically or cost-effective.

The task is potentially enormous. Clinical practice variations are endemic in the Health Service[6] and NICE will have a relatively small budget (£9 million) with which to tackle this challenging remit.

Since it will only be able to scratch the surface of the problem, the selection of technologies for formal appraisal by NICE assumes considerable importance. This is to be decided by a special committee within the Department of Health. The emphasis will be on clinical innovations or new technologies that could have significant clinical or cost impact on the NHS, and on existing technologies where there are 'unexplained' or 'unacceptable' variations in use or 'uncertainty about clinical effectiveness or cost-effectiveness'.[5] Current proposals for criteria for choosing which technologies should be appraised are summarised in Box 2.

BOX 2: SUGGESTED CRITERIA FOR SELECTING PRIORITIES FOR APPRAISING HEALTH TECHNOLOGIES[3]

1. What is the total potential cost to the NHS of using the intervention to treat the condition for which it is intended?
2. What is the maximum likely benefit (including non-NHS benefits) of treating the condition?
3. What will be the impact on non-financial NHS resources, i.e. on staff and infrastructure, of introducing the technology?
4. What are the likely consequences on resource use of not issuing guidance on appropriate use of the technology?
5. Will this technology create new expectations and demands?
6. Are the effects of this technology likely to remain controversial?
7. Are there any relevant ethical concerns?
8. Is there any doubt about whether this technology is appropriate for NHS funding?
9. In the case of an existing technology, is there controversy over best practice and are there wide variations in practice patterns?

Presumably the Department's committee will not be expected to have the answers to these questions – that is the task of the appraisal process. Selection will therefore be based on expert opinion about the likely significance of a particular innovation or existing treatment in relation to these criteria. If members of the NICE appraisal committee are to produce recommendations that have a reasonable chance of being adopted by health authorities and clinicians, they will need to find the answers to this list of questions. Thus, they will need access to detailed evidence for each of the selected health technologies: on clinical outcomes; on costs, risks and benefits; on the likely impact on non-financial resource use; on associated non-NHS costs, for example personal social services costs; on patients' expectations and likely demands; on the views of clinicians, ethicists, politicians and the public.

NICE will adopt a seven-stage process to appraise new technologies (Box 3):

BOX 3: NICE APPRAISAL PROCESS

1. Manufacturer invited to submit data to support appraisal four to six months before launch
2. Manufacturer submits dossier
3. Data evaluated by NICE secretariat
4. Manufacturer's data and secretariat's evaluation considered by appraisal committee
5. Draft appraisal report published, seeking the views of the manufacturer, professional and patient organisations, and the Department of Health
6. Appraisal committee reviews advice and submits final appraisal report to the Board of NICE
7. NICE releases report

For new technologies, the plan is to rely on the manufacturer or commercial sponsor to provide the evidence for use in the appraisal. The licensing process overseen by the Medicines Control Agency requires companies to provide data on the quality, safety and efficacy of new drugs, so this information should be readily available for use in NICE appraisals. Such data will not be so easily obtained for medical devices, diagnostic instruments or surgical procedures, which do not at present have to undergo such rigorous scrutiny before they are introduced into the NHS. Even for drugs, however, current requirements do not include provision of evidence on cost-effectiveness or on the longer-term effects of the treatment. Assessments of efficacy are usually based on a limited number of clinical indicators; length of outcomes follow-up is often very short and drug trials rarely include measures of the impact of the treatment on the patient's quality of life or on NHS resource use.

For new technologies it will be virtually impossible to gather much of this evidence within the tight timescale set for the appraisal process (about seven months). Relevant information may be generated via the health technology assessment strand of the NHS research and development programme for certain existing treatments, but in the initial stages of NICE's work this is only likely to be available in a few instances. The Association of the British Pharmaceutical Industry (ABPI) has argued that assessment of cost-effectiveness and value for money cannot be determined reliably until a new therapy has been in use in the general population for some time.[7]

Thus it seems certain that the appraisal committee will have to base their recommendations on economic modelling – an imprecise art – backed up by their informed judgements and forecasts. They will nevertheless be expected to produce clear and precise recommendations, summarised into one of three categories:

- recommended as clinically cost-effective for routine use in the NHS or only for particular patient subgroups
- recommended only for use in the context of clinical trials to help answer specific questions about cost-effectiveness or targeting
- not recommended for routine use.

The NICE Board will therefore find themselves in a similar position to anyone else who has tried to devise evidence-based recommendations or guidelines – the evidence is necessarily incomplete and insufficiently reliable to eliminate the need for judgement.[8] Even expert opinion can vary when it comes to devising guidelines, and the most careful consensus development procedures cannot rule out the possibility that different groups of experts will arrive at different conclusions after scrutinising the same data. NICE should expect to receive challenges from groups or individuals who disagree with their recommendations.

If the NICE recommendations or guidelines are to have a chance of commanding widespread support, they must be as scientifically rigorous as possible and the basis for the judgements must be very clearly stated. This means making the research available for public scrutiny and being clear about gaps in the evidence and the value base underlying the committee's recommendations. This level of transparency is unlikely to be willingly complied with by the manufacturers, who may wish to keep their research data confidential to avoid making it available to competitors. At the same time the companies are likely to vigorously challenge any recommendations that do not concur with their estimate of the value of their products. These challenges may be hard to defend if the evidence on which they are based is not in the public domain. The NICE appraisal committee will have to balance the demands of the sponsors to treat the data they submit as 'commercial in confidence' against the need for public scrutiny of the basis of their recommendations.

Political problems

Media interest in 'postcode prescribing' has centred on patients denied access to specific high-cost treatments such as interferon beta for multiple sclerosis, taxol for breast cancer, aricept for Alzheimer's disease, and *in vitro* fertilisation to treat infertility. Denial of these treatments to certain groups of patients on the basis of non-clinical criteria such as where they happen to live has been seen (correctly) as an example of rationing in action. Health authorities under pressure to meet budget targets have made different decisions about which expensive treatments they will pay for. Press stories about patients in neighbouring authorities apparently having different entitlements to treatment have proved shocking to a public accustomed to thinking about the NHS as a fair and equitable service.

The media is interested in this issue in part because it provides a rich source of human interest stories, but also because journalists perceive hypocrisy in the statements of ministers and senior officials who deny that rationing occurs in the NHS. Rationing is the process of choosing which beneficial services should be offered to whom, and which should not.[9] It is, and always has been, a feature of health care delivery in every country, but successive British governments have been reluctant to admit to its existence. If the NHS had access to unlimited resources, rationing would not be an issue, but a service that has to operate within budget limits cannot avoid the need to make hard choices. Government spokesmen prefer to talk about priority-setting – a less alarming phrase, which serves to obscure the fact that access to some potentially beneficial treatments or services has to be restricted. Mechanisms for rationing include *denial* of treatment, *selection* by restricting treatments to particular groups, *deflection* to a different service, *deterrence* by raising barriers to access, *delay* through queues or waiting lists, *dilution* by restricting the quantity or quality of care, or *termination* by early discharge from treatment.[10]

In establishing NICE, the Government has acknowledged the need for a more rational and transparent mechanism for deciding on priorities, but this process cannot be value-free. Decisions about the allocation of health care resources can, and should, be based on sound evidence about the potential benefit derived from particular treatments and the cost of providing them, but making these choices depends on values as well as technical evidence. The decision about whether or not to allocate resources to a particular treatment or service involves consideration of whether it is *affordable*, in relation to other calls on funds, and whether it is an *appropriate* use of taxpayers' money. 'Rational' rationing requires a consensus on the objectives and scope of the NHS (for example, is it appropriate for a public service to treat impotence or infertility?) and on the desired outcomes of medical treatment. There has to be agreement on the relative importance of the various goals of the service and on how its performance should be measured. In making choices between competing demands on resources one has to decide whose values should be taken into account (those of the public, patients, carers, user groups, clinicians, managers, politicians?) and who should be the final arbiter when these values conflict.

On scrutinising the list in Box 2 it is clear that in addition to the 'technical' criteria of quality, safety and efficacy, issues of affordability and appropriateness will inevitably come into play in making recommendations. The Government's guidelines on drug treatments for impotence[11] were issued prior to the establishment of NICE, but they illustrate the case well. Viagra is an effective drug, which has considerable advantages over existing treatments for impotence, but the Government decided to restrict its use to certain groups of patients (i.e. to ration it) because of concern about its potential impact on the NHS budget (i.e. its *affordability*). This decision was influenced by doubts, shared by many clinicians and members of the public, about the *appropriateness* of treating impotence on the NHS. Thus, despite protests from the manufacturer of this drug and from some clinicians and patients, it was possible to discern a significant constituency of support for the decision to restrict its availability.

In making this decision, the Government's advisers had to consider the position from the point of view of the competing interests involved, i.e. the patients who might benefit from the drug, the clinicians who might wish to give their patients this effective treatment, the drug company that would benefit from maximising sales of the drug, the health authorities that would have to pay for it out of their patient care budgets, other patients who might have to forgo treatments if resources were used up in treating impotence, and the public who may or may not feel that this was a good use of taxpayers' money.

However much the Government may want to present the appraisal of new treatments and technologies as a purely technical process to be consigned to expert committees, it is clear that decisions about affordability and appropriateness are political issues that should be open to public scrutiny and debate. In the case of Viagra the responsibility for weighing the balance between these competing interests lay on the shoulders of the Secretary of State for Health. This is entirely appropriate since he or she is accountable to Parliament for Health Service expenditure, but for many less high-profile treatments the decisions have in the past been left to local budgetholders, i.e. the health authorities. It is this devolution of financial and policy responsibility that has led to postcode prescribing. There is nothing in the Government's published plans to suggest that this local discretion will not be allowed to continue. The Government may be hoping that all health authorities and PCGs will follow NICE guidance to the letter, but there is no guarantee that this will happen. The mere existence of national guidelines may not be sufficient to ensure that variations are eliminated.

There will be a high level of interest in NICE's recommendations, especially among those who stand to gain or lose most, i.e. the health care industry and patients. It will be very important for NICE to ensure that its decision-making processes are as transparent as possible. The organisation will need to become an effective player in the political arena in which it will inevitably find itself, but the boundaries between NICE and the Department of Health will have to be carefully drawn. A committee of unelected and unaccountable experts is not an appropriate body to decide between competing interests, but they could be given responsibility for developing a framework for decision-making and for overseeing public consultation. Ultimately, rationing decisions should remain the explicit responsibility of elected representatives. This means the Government must acknowledge the fact of rationing. If it took this step it could claim considerable credit for establishing NICE as the first stage in a more rational system for ensuring the fair allocation of resources. Without this acknowledgement NICE will be left with an impossible task.

THE COMMISSION FOR HEALTH IMPROVEMENT

The CHI has been established as an independent statutory body directly accountable to the Secretary of State. At the time of writing plans for CHI were still sketchy. Its stated remit includes five main functions:[3]

- to provide national leadership to develop and disseminate clinical governance principles
- to scrutinise local clinical governance arrangements through a rolling programme of local reviews of NHS trusts and primary care trusts
- to monitor implementation of national service frameworks and NICE guidance
- to help the NHS identify and tackle serious or persistent clinical problems and to act as a trouble-shooter to put things right
- to oversee and assist with external incident enquiries.

The precise nature of the relationship between CHI and organisations such as the regional offices of the NHS Executive, health authorities and PCGs, the Royal Colleges and other professional regulatory bodies, the Audit Commission, the Health and Safety Executive, the Social Services Inspectorate and NICE, is not yet clear. The regional offices have responsibility for monitoring performance in health authorities and trusts, including the development of clinical governance and implementation of NICE guidance and the national service frameworks. *A First Class Service* states that CHI 'will not replace mainstream

NHS performance assessment and management, but will complement and reinforce these processes'.[3] Precisely how it will do this is not yet clear. CHI could perhaps facilitate national co-ordination of this work and act as an external regulator to monitor and develop the effectiveness of self-regulation carried out by the professional bodies. It is also intended that CHI should act as a trouble-shooter, being ready to investigate problems when invited to do so by the regional offices. The Board of CHI will have to ensure that it devotes sufficient time to developing and managing potentially difficult relationships with professional organisations.

The Commission will have three main responsibilities: to identify problems and poor clinical standards, to develop quality improvement systems, and to oversee the implementation of national clinical standards. None of these tasks is going to be straightforward.

Identifying problems

How will CHI or the regional offices identify quality problems? Some information will be available routinely through the national performance framework.[12] This includes indicators of performance in relation to six dimensions:

- health improvement
- fair access
- effective delivery of appropriate health care
- efficiency
- patient/carer experience
- health outcomes.

When these indicators were published in full for the first time,[13] they were widely reported in the press in the form of league tables with comments about 'the best' and 'the worst' hospitals in relation to specific indices, usually mortality rates. Clinicians and managers in the trusts at the bottom of the league immediately claimed the data were inaccurate or incomplete and misrepresented the true situation in their hospitals. In many cases these claims had some justification, since data quality is known to be poor in a number of areas. The figures were not adjusted for case-mix, so could not make allowance for problems due to a hospital's difficult caseload rather than to an inherent quality failure. A low position in the league table may be an indication of a possible problem, but if the trouble-shooters are sent in on the basis of these data alone, trusts may be tempted to massage their figures or be more selective about their caseload in order to move up the league.

A common criticism of formal systems for monitoring quality is that they fall into the trap of measuring the easily measurable and ignore the less tangible but sometimes more important aspects of health care. There is very little agreement on the most valid and useful quality indicators and no consensus about the most important goals of quality improvement.[14] The patient survey will provide a new source of data, which may prove to be a more useful indicator of the quality of clinical care than those available hitherto, but this is as yet untested. *A First Class Service* states that CHI's review teams will have access to 'individual clinician's external clinical audit results'[3] (para.4.12). This points to much closer external scrutiny of clinical work than has ever been the case before, but it is suggestive of an approach that is geared towards looking for 'bad apples' rather than one which is primarily aimed at developing quality improvement processes.

Promoting quality improvements

Recent experience of clinical audit programmes demonstrates the problems that must be avoided if clinical governance is to have a real impact. Many clinical audit projects were nothing more than data-gathering exercises or poor-quality research projects. There were few sanctions against clinicians who did not want to participate and managers were only infrequently involved. It was rare to find a hospital that had a clear, organisation-wide strategy for promoting clinical audit and a mechanism for ensuring that it led to real quality improvements.

There is a natural tendency to look for scapegoats when evidence of bad practice emerges, but quality failures can rarely be pinpointed to the action of a few individuals. More often they are the result of a system failure in which processes to assure quality were not in place or were not working properly. It follows, then, that CHI should concentrate on system-wide solutions if it is to make a real impact on quality improvement. A recent national experiment using a multifaceted approach to raise clinical quality standards demonstrated the potential scope of a system-wide approach to clinical governance.[15] The Promoting Action on Clinical Effectiveness (PACE) programme supported changes in clinical practice in 16 sites around the country. The experiences of the programme suggest that trusts need to have systems in place to:

- enable clinical staff to routinely review the quality of clinical practice
- ensure that standards for care are established and implemented
- ensure that patients are at the centre of work that develops and monitors local standards
- ensure that the implementation of change is managed effectively
- support the development of individuals and clinical teams through a systematic approach to education and training.

This points to the need to integrate quality improvement into all aspects of the organisation's work. It is intended that the Commission should work with trusts in cases where there are 'serious or persistent problems ... [to] both investigate and identify the source of the problem, and work with the organisation on lasting remedies' (para.4.2).[3] It is doubtful that this organisational development task will sit easily alongside the roles of inspector and external regulator.

Implementing national standards

If the Government's goal of reducing practice variations is to be achieved, it will require more than the publication of national standards and guidelines. Changing clinical practice is a complex task requiring multifaceted interventions that target specific barriers to change.[16] Strategies to change practice need to be adequately resourced and led by people with appropriate knowledge and skills. It is not clear where this investment will come from. Trust boards will have formal responsibility for ensuring that change does happen, but they will have to manage this within their current level of resources. With about 400 trusts to review and support over the course of a three- to four-year rolling programme, and with a budget of only £3 million, CHI will be hard pressed to make much of an impact on its own. It might be able to spread the load by building effective alliances with the professional bodies, but these relationships could be easily damaged if CHI adopts a top-down or coercive approach to quality improvement, which relies on 'naming and shaming'.

It is too early to see where, in practice, the balance will lie between self-directed or bottom-up systems for quality improvement and centrally directed, top-down approaches. The debate about which is most likely to achieve results centres on the relative merits of facilitative or participative approaches to quality improvement, which rely on staff involvement and personal commitment, versus more coercive approaches that emphasise externally imposed incentives and sanctions. Current accepted wisdom prefers the carrot to the stick in the belief that quality is not best served by a climate of fear.[17] The problem is that methods that depend on voluntary involvement can be ignored by those whose practices give most cause for concern. It seems likely that a combination of carrot and stick is required, but what is the optimal balance? Despite the extensive experience of quality improvement processes in the public sector, in industry and commerce, and in health care systems around the world, there has been very little rigorous comparative research that could settle the argument. In the light of this uncertainty the Government has, perhaps wisely, set out a programme which could encompass both coercive and facilitative models.

The mere existence of a national body such as CHI does not necessarily imply a move towards coercion. In theory there is no reason why it could not evolve into a development agency which leads and facilitates locally based quality improvement programmes, but the indications are that its role as inspector will take precedence over a more developmental function. The reasons for this lie in the Government's determination to root out poor practice and to provide a counterweight to existing systems of self-regulation, the shortcomings of which became starkly apparent during the Bristol case.[18] The risk is that undue emphasis on what Taylor calls 'zero tolerance of failure'[17] will lead to conflict and fear among staff instead of empowering them to cope with the difficult challenges they face.

CONCLUSION

In distinguishing its approach from the previous government's attempts to promote diversity and market competition as the driver for quality improvement, the present Government has laid much greater stress on centrally controlled mechanisms for raising standards. The two newly established national institutions, NICE and CHI, can be seen as the embodiment of the shift towards a centralised approach to standard-setting and quality improvement in England and Wales. Time will tell whether these organisations can command sufficient respect from the various stakeholders to successfully lead the drive to improve standards of clinical care and rebuild public confidence in the NHS.

REFERENCES

1. Secretary of State for Health. *The New NHS: modern, dependable*. London: The Stationery Office, 1997.

2. Maxwell R. Dimensions of quality revisited: from thought to action. *Quality in Health Care* 1992; 1: 171–77.

3. Department of Health. *A first class service: quality in The New NHS*. London: Department of Health, 1998.

4. Rawlins M. In pursuit of quality: the National Institute for Clinical Excellence. *Lancet* 1999; 353: 1079–82.

5. NHS Executive. *Faster access to modern treatment: how NICE appraisal will work*. NHSE, 1999.

6. Andersen TF, Mooney G. *The challenges of medical practice variations*. London: Macmillan Press, 1990.

7. ABPI. *NICE and medicines*. Leaflet BSC/6/99/4k. June 1999.

8. Woolf SH, Grol R, Hutchinson A, Eccles M, Grimshaw J. Potential benefits, limitations and harms of clinical guidelines. *BMJ* 1999; 318: 527–30.

9. New B. *The rationing agenda in the NHS*. London: King's Fund, 1996.

10. Klein R, Day P, Redmayne S. *Managing scarcity*. Milton Keynes: Open University Press, 1996.

11. NHS Executive. *Treatment for impotence*. Health Service Circular 1999/115. NHSE, 1999.

12. NHS Executive. *The New NHS modern and dependable: a national framework for assessing performance*. Executive Letter (98) 4.

13. NHS Executive. *Quality and performance in the NHS: high level performance indicators*. NHSE, 1999.

14. Greenhalgh T, Eversley J. *Quality in general practice*. London: King's Fund, 1999.

15. Dunning M, Abi-Aad G, Gilbert D, Hutton H, Brown C. *Experience, evidence and everyday practice*. London: King's Fund, 1999.

16. NHS Centre for Reviews and Dissemination. Getting evidence into practice. *Effective Health Care* 1999; 5: 1.

17. Taylor, D. *Improving health care*. London: King's Fund, 1998.

18. Klein R. Competence, professional self-regulation, and the public interest. *BMJ* 1998; 316: 1740–1742.

Rationing access to elective care: the way forward

Waiting lists refuse to come down: a fresh approach is required.

Anthony Harrison and Bill New

Since its foundation, the NHS has been rationing access to elective hospital care. Nevertheless, it has not developed a principled approach to this task. Instead, it has allowed the rationing process to be managed by individual clinicians, following their own judgements as to whom to treat and what order to treat people in.

In this respect, elective hospital care is no different from any other part of the NHS. In other respects, however, elective care is different: in the first place, the total numbers of people waiting for elective care have been regularly published, so although the process of rationing has been implicit, the existence of rationing has been apparent. Moreover, throughout most of the post-war period, but with increasing emphasis during the 1990s, successive governments have actively attempted to reduce either the time spent waiting or the numbers waiting, or both – measures which work to reduce the impact of the rationing effect. Despite these measures, numbers waiting have continued to grow to well over 1 million.

In this article, we:

- set out how we believe elective care is rationed, i.e. how waiting affects the level of access
- describe the policies adopted by the Labour Government and show why they are inadequate
- set out two alternative policies, one radical and one incremental.

HOW RATIONING WORKS

Although it has been acknowledged for 20 years or more that waiting lists perform a rationing function, the way they do so is rarely made clear. The critical question is how exactly does waiting affect patients' access to care?

The pathway to elective care is set out in Figure 1. In this simplified depiction of the process, there are three decision-makers:

- the patient
- the GP
- the specialist.

Each may be influenced by the length of the wait the patient may have to experience, but in different ways.

FIGURE 1

ELECTIVE CARE: ACCESS STAGES

Stage 1: Perceive illness and decide to seek medical advice
Visit GP

Stage 2: GP consultation: decision on referral
Refer to out-patient consultation

Stage 3: Consultant diagnosis: decision to place on waiting list
Place on waiting list

Stage 4: Consultant decision on admission for treatment
Treatment: health outcome

At each stage, decisions have to be made by different actors. Typically, patients gain access to elective care by seeking advice from their GP (stage 1) and then passing through the next three stages if the professionals – GPs and consultants – agree that treatment is appropriate. Alternatively, the patient may decide to 'live with' their condition and not seek treatment. The GP may advise, or decide on behalf of the patient, that an alternative treatment strategy, e.g. of an ameliorative kind, may be preferable to a long wait. The consultant may decide that the patient's condition is not far enough advanced to merit treatment and defer the decision to accept the patient on to the list to some future date. In all these cases, a decision is being made that there is little to be gained by the patients being placed on a waiting list, despite the apparent need for care. Waiting therefore reduces, in an informal and inexplicit way, the number of 'low value' claims on NHS resources; but the judgement as to what is 'low value' is made in different ways along the care path.

If delay does affect the three decision-makers in these ways, then any attempt to reduce *time* spent waiting will have the effect of increasing the *numbers* joining the queue. Waiting, in other words, acts as a proxy for price. As with prices in other markets, there will be some who are unresponsive to changes in waiting times – those who do not mind waiting or who do mind but are undeterred by it because they are determined to be treated. But if no one were deterred, then there would be no rationing effect. People would be delayed, but still gain treatment in the end. Access is controlled, but not rationed.

Waiting within the NHS may ration in a further way. In the early 1990s, the concept of a 'mortlake' was set out by Frankel & West.[1] They used this term to describe the existence of people on the list whose priority was never going to be high enough for them to be treated but whose condition – e.g. varicose veins – was recognised as being treatable. In effect, their claims for treatment were constantly being pushed back by the identification of more urgent or valuable claims. However, with the introduction of maximum waiting times in the Patient's Charter, the mortlake was abolished, since anyone put on a waiting list has been more or less guaranteed treatment within a specified time.

There is no rationing effect where patients divert to the private sector. Those able to divert because they are privately insured or are able to pay may be seeking nearly any elective procedure. Whether this effect is desirable or not involves an equity judgement. In some health systems, e.g. Canada, it is not allowed precisely because the ability to queue jump in this way is seen as running counter to the overall system's aims. In the UK, the Government, despite its commitment to equity and its rejection of queue jumping by GP fundholding patients, has turned a blind eye to this escape route from rationing.

If this were the whole story, then the increase in the volume of elective care observed since the beginning of the NHS would have meant that the additional resources that the NHS has devoted to it would be yielding less and less value: the proportion of non-serious conditions would have risen and the thresholds at which progressive conditions are treated would have fallen.

But other forces have been at work, of which probably the most important has been progress in medical technology, which has both introduced new procedures and enabled them to be applied to an ever increasing proportion of the population. This has meant that new 'high value' activity – procedures such as joint replacement and cataract removal – have prevented the 'market' for elective care being exhausted by the higher levels of activity and led to procedures which are widely regarded as being effective in removing disability.

FIGURE 2

TECHNICAL CHANGE AND ACCESS THRESHOLDS

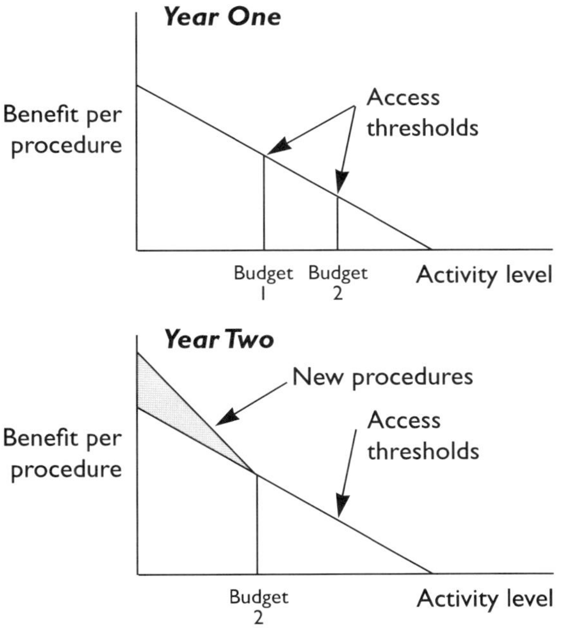

Thus, on the top section of Figure 2, we show the implications of expanding the volume of elective activity, assuming no change in technology. The volume of activity rises and the access threshold falls as patients with less serious conditions gain access. In the lower part, the shaded area represents new procedures made possible by technical progress that are assumed to be of high value. To simplify the diagram, it has been drawn so that the new procedures require budget level 2, which cannot now be used to finance the lower value activity lying between budget limits 1 and 2 on the left-hand side. As a result, the threshold for entry to care remains the same, even though the budget has risen.

The 'price', mortlake and new technology effects go a long way to explaining key features of waiting lists within the NHS:

- the total numbers identified for treatment have risen while activity has also risen
- specific initiatives to reduce numbers waiting, such as the Conservatives' waiting time initiative, had an initial impact but failed to dent the upward trend
- some people, until the Patient's Charter limits were introduced in 1991, waited for extremely long periods even though the majority of patients were seen quickly.

NEW LABOUR

The policies adopted by the new Government consist of two main strands:

- a short-term element, with the emphasis on reducing numbers waiting and setting maximum waiting times
- a longer-term element, with the emphasis on national standards of performance across the country as a whole, which, if realised, should provide everyone with a similar standard of service and access.

The first element has been widely criticised, largely on the ground that numbers waiting are not important, but access times are, and that it is possible, as experience in the 1990s has demonstrated, for access times to fall while numbers waiting increase. Furthermore, the fact that waiting occurs at an earlier stage in the process of gaining access to care, particularly in the period between referral and being seen at an out-patient clinic, has been made public since figures began to be collected in 1995. The latest figures suggest that numbers waiting at this stage have been rising more or less in line with the fall in numbers waiting for admission that has taken place since late 1997.

But there are further, and hitherto less emphasised, weaknesses.

First, the national total has no significance in itself. NHS waiting lists vary from one part of the country to another. The existence of differences in the size of waiting lists and access times between different parts of the country implies that the outcome of the rationing process is different in different parts of the country, even if the broad forces at work are the same. Whether this matters or not depends on the value placed on equity and on the reasons underlying these variations. Some may be regarded as reflecting 'local choice', others as (undesirable) differences in clinical effectiveness and operational efficiency between different parts of the hospital system.

Given the scale of variation between areas – at all stages of the access process – this mix is likely to vary a great deal from one part of the country to another. As noted already, while that could reflect local choice – be it of health authority or individual surgeon – it also reflects variations in hospital staffing and the availability of physical facilities as well as professional uncertainties about 'what works'.

This is where the second strand of the Government's policy comes into play. In *The New NHS* and *A First Class Service* it set outs its intention, supported by the national performance assessment framework and national service frameworks, to reduce variations in the standard of care offered in different parts of the country and variations in the efficiency of service delivery. Although not specifically targeted at waiting lists, these measures will tend to reduce variations in access to elective care between different parts of the country.

Secondly, short lists may reflect poor performance in primary care as much as good performance in secondary. The waiting list only shows those whose need for treatment has been identified. But there is evidence that the needs of many people are not identified, even when they consult their GP. For example, in line with an earlier study in the same field, a recent National Audit Office study of cataract surgery found that many patients were reaching hospital at an advanced stage of the disease, beyond the thresholds the hospitals themselves were using when deciding whether to accept someone for treatment.[2] As a recent *BMJ* editorial noted:

> *Achieving optimal outcomes from cataract surgery is not as simple as merely reducing waiting times but must also focus on ensuring the early identification and prioritisation of patients at risk of functional decline and dependency due to visual symptoms.*[3]

This puts the emphasis on primary care services – including patients themselves – rather than the hospital service.

Thirdly, the numbers waiting for treatment give no guidance as to what level of resources should be devoted to elective care, i.e. how the total 'ration' should be determined. Taken to its extreme, the Government's policy of targeting numbers waiting would lead to the abolition of waiting altogether. But while waiting for access to elective care scarcely exists in high-spending health care countries, it persists in other countries that spend more on health care than England – such as Canada and Sweden, and Scotland, which spends nearly a quarter more per head than England – and is beginning to emerge in high-spending countries such as Germany. Elimination of waiting lists does not seem feasible so the total budget for elective care must be determined by reference to some other criterion. By implication, the present Government's target of 100,000 fewer people waiting than the number when it came to office provides that criterion – except that it is only too obvious that this number is arbitrary and has no justification in its own right.

Even if it were feasible to eliminate all waiting, it would not necessarily be desirable. If the Government continues to expand the health care budget in the hope of removing the numbers recorded as waiting, and if the mechanics work as we suggest, more and more patients will come forward for treatment. Some will come from the private sector, with serious conditions but now finding the wait for NHS treatment tolerable; others will come from all sources, but with less serious complaints.

While there may well be a case for expanding elective activity in areas such as joint replacement, where cost and clinical effectiveness appear to be high, the general case for doing so has not been made. If gains from further activity decline, as suggested in Figure 2 above, then at some point a line must be drawn. Otherwise the benefits of spending more would be less than their value in other health uses or other public spending programmes.

At the present time, the basis for making any judgement on what the budget should be is absent. Although the Government has devoted extra, targeted resources to the reduction of waiting lists, it has no means at its disposal of determining what extra activity – in terms of its composition – it is getting in return. However, there is a case for reducing waiting times.

Until the recent National User Survey, there had been no official survey of people's attitudes towards waiting since the Royal Commission in the 1970s. Both have shown that waiting is not a cause of distress or additional pain for some people, but that it is for a significant number of others.

TABLE 1

WHETHER CONDITION WORSENED BEFORE BEING SEEN

Male			*Age*		
%	*Under 25*	*25–34*	*35–44*	*45–64*	*65+*
A little worse	34	25	28	29	29
A lot worse	8	8	9	8	5
Stayed the same/got better	49	57	51	54	51
Not sure	9	10	12	9	15
Unweighted	357	797	1089	2989	2465
Weighted	644	1440	1309	2665	1905

Female			*Age*		
%	*Under 25*	*25–34*	*35–44*	*45–64*	*65+*
A little worse	31	23	23	30	30
A lot worse	7	7	8	7	8
Stayed the same/got better	50	55	58	53	48
Not sure	12	15	11	10	14
Unweighted	684	1633	1980	3879	2831
Weighted	861	1943	1769	2985	2439

Source: National survey of NHS patients: General Practice 1998. London: Department of Health, 1999.

TABLE 2

WHETHER CONDITION CAUSED PAIN

Male			*Age*		
%	*Under 25*	*25–34*	*35–44*	*45–64*	*65+*
Lots of pain	13	14	16	15	10
Some pain	46	45	45	41	38
Not in pain	38	38	37	43	50
Cannot remember	3	3	2	1	2
Unweighted	354	795	1088	2978	2460
Weighted	638	1435	1308	2655	1901

Female			*Age*		
%	*Under 25*	*25–34*	*35–44*	*45–64*	*65+*
Lots of pain	13	12	13	16	17
Some pain	36	33	37	41	39
Not in pain	48	53	48	41	41
Cannot remember	3	2	2	2	3
Unweighted	682	1630	1984	3879	2845
Weighted	859	1940	1774	2985	2453

Source: National survey of NHS patients: General Practice 1998. London: Department of Health, 1999.

These data are an insufficient basis for determining what waits are reasonable for what conditions, but the aim of eliminating all waiting where the wait itself is painful or imposes other serious costs on patients – and their carers – would have a *prima facie* justification. The same is true where waiting is risky in terms of mortality and an increased risk of poor outcome. As we have shown elsewhere,[4] evidence of the clinical significance of delay is patchy and inconclusive, but recent studies of waiting for coronary artery bypass grafts (CABGs) suggest a significant level of mortality while patients are awaiting treatment.[5]

OVERALL

Waiting for access to elective care performs an essential rationing function, by deterring some potential users from seeking treatment or professionals from offering it. The current Government's emphasis on cutting numbers may fail in its own terms if, as past experience as well as current figures suggest, more people come forward for treatment. However, if it succeeds, it provides no means of determining how much should be allocated to elective care, how that budget should be shared among the various competing claims upon it and how the claims themselves should be identified. Furthermore, the process by which claims are made on the existing budget is largely implicit and, in critical areas, based on poor information.

BROAD POLICY OPTIONS

We have argued that waiting lists perform an essential function – that of rationing access to care – but:

- they may be inefficient, in the sense that they do not necessarily lead to the best possible mix of elective care being provided, particularly when they are combined with maximum waits regardless of the condition to be treated
- they may be inequitable between people with

FIGURE 3

ACCESS AND THE PRIORITY THRESHOLD

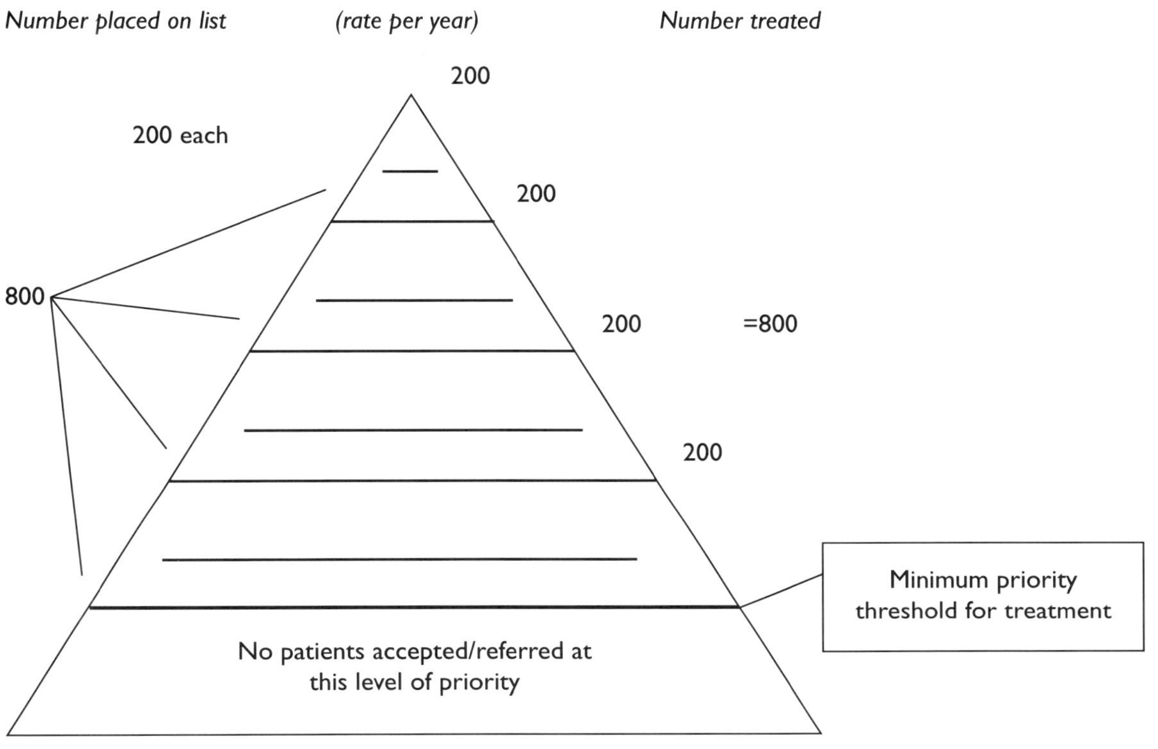

- the same condition in different areas and between people with different conditions
- the way they currently work – i.e. the order in which patients are treated – is obscure and 'unaccountable'
- they undoubtedly impose costs on those waiting, but there has been very little research on the extent of these costs, or the precise circumstances within which they arise.

The question we consider in this section is whether access to elective care can be rationed in a more efficient, equitable and accountable manner.

A SCORE-BASED WAITING SYSTEM

We first set out a radical option, based on experience in New Zealand. The key technical element in this approach is the definition of thresholds, which patients must 'jump' before they can gain access to publicly funded care. It is the threshold – or set of thresholds – that carries out the rationing function, not the long waiting times. This system, in broad outline, works as follows.

Figure 3 represents flows of patients with conditions of different degrees of severity. Instead of the development of a mortlake consisting of all those patients who will never be treated, or have a very low likelihood of being treated, a priority threshold is introduced, determined by the provider's treatment capacity (either a local NHS trust or the NHS as a whole). Those with conditions which do not 'score' sufficiently to cross this threshold are told that they cannot be treated because there are insufficient public resources for their level of 'need'. They are returned to primary care for management and may return if their condition becomes more serious. Those who satisfy the threshold criteria are guaranteed treatment within a given period, the precise time depending on their level of priority.

In fact, two lines are drawn. The first is a 'clinical threshold', determined by an assessment of the clinical factors which would 'ideally' indicate to a clinician that treatment should take place. The second is the 'financial threshold', below which people are referred back and which is determined by the level of finance available for elective treatment. Not surprisingly, there is typically a gap between the two, with the clinical lower than the financial (otherwise the 'normal' clinical decision-making would be enough to bring the system into balance). In fact, it is unlikely that the clinical threshold is actually objective: it probably reflects in part the context of financial constraints and medical norms. There is also an incentive to pitch it at a politically realistic level, thereby encouraging politicians to raise the financial threshold until it matches the clinical. Such clinical thresholds, however, have a habit of becoming moving targets, i.e. adapting to the prevailing financial climate.

Waiting lists are not abolished, but they are organised to include only those for whom treatment can be guaranteed within a given period. There is no need for a mortlake, or sheer list size, to act as a deterrent: maximum waits are defined, but only for conditions that are judged to deserve reasonably rapid treatment.

What this period should be is matter of judgement. At first sight it may not be necessary: the initial assessment of a lower threshold score is calculated specifically to match supply to demand. Thus, the rate of acceptance for treatment will be the same as that for treatment itself – the system will be in equilibrium. In theory, then, there is no need for any waiting: with perfect information, patients with scores above the threshold could be treated immediately.

However, information is not perfect and there is always some unpredictable variability in demand. A maximum six-month lead-in to treatment was chosen in New Zealand as a reasonable compromise between the system being too 'tight' and inflexible, and too 'loose', with bookings taken too far ahead and thus liable to cancellation. In practice, the system approximates to the triangle in Figure 3: high-priority patients at the top are treated within a month; low-priority patients, but above the threshold, are treated within six months.

The system just described brings with it a whole range of issues that are as yet unresolved – even in New Zealand where the system is successfully operating in localised forms. The first set of issues relates to equity. Systems for determining clinical scores have been developed locally and thus vary from area to area, potentially leaving identical patients with different priority scores and thus different chances of treatment. These variations reflect the fact that very little work has been done world-wide on what such scoring systems should comprise and what the relative waits of the various elements should be. In the UK, there have been only a few experiments, typically within a given specialty. And, as noted above, for the majority of conditions there is very little data about the risks of postponing treatment, the effect of delay on outcome and the pain and other costs patients suffer while waiting.

To make comparisons *between* disease groups or specialties requires *generic* scoring systems comprising elements common to all conditions, but these have not yet been developed. Some degree of generic scoring is also needed properly to prioritise *within* certain waiting list categories: between different surgical orthopaedic procedures, for example, or for cardiac surgery. Finally, the greater the need to choose between cases requiring different interventions (even within a particular surgical specialty), the more salient the issue of cost becomes. If it is not incorporated as a potential scoring criterion – and the New Zealand system leaves it out – then it will be impossible to maximise the aggregate benefit for a given waiting list (unless cases are very similar in cost terms, as with cataract surgery). Clinicians are often reluctant to incorporate cost, seeing it as an unwelcome intrusion of economics into their sphere of activity. But, within a fixed budget, financial cost acts as a measure of the claims of other patients to treatment and this, the opportunity cost, is clearly relevant to making the best of a given budget.

Over and above these technical issues, there are other difficulties. The system will increase pressure on health care professionals. Primary care practitioners will have to explain why publicly financed treatment is being denied (if only temporarily). This will be a difficult task since GPs will have to balance their desire to provide care for the individual with the imperatives of the system. Should they encourage people who can afford it to use the private sector? Should they encourage those whose prognosis is predictable (and thus will cross the financial threshold at a given point in the future) to return at that date, building up future pressures, or leave it to the patient to decide? Will GPs go along with it or simply reject any such policy and disrupt it from within, perhaps by repeatedly sending back patients for assessment and clogging-up out-patient clinics?

The effect on the NHS budget could go either way. The perceived gap between clinical and financial thresholds could provide pressure on the Treasury to increase spending. On the other hand, if the cases referred back are perceived to be of low 'value' socially (and if many of these cases make greater use of the private sector), pressure on spending may be mitigated. Whichever way the balance goes, the identification of cut-offs and, hence, shortfalls provides the basis for debate about how much should be spent on elective care.

The effect on public opinion is also highly uncertain. Will the public accept the new political 'contract', or will it reject public provision in favour of the private sector? The answer to this depends on precisely what is valued in a publicly financed health system. Is it, on the one hand, its (apparently) all-inclusive nature and the external benefits this provides in terms of reassurance, social solidarity and sense of community? Or is it, on the other hand, its ability to provide the maximum benefit for those who have the most pressing claims, regardless of ability to pay, in a reliable, predictable and democratically accountable way? Again this is a debate which has not yet been effectively joined in the UK.

Overall, the system described here is essentially based on a belief in openness and honesty about what a health care system can achieve under budget constraints in return for a genuine degree of certainty about when treatment will occur. The political 'deal' it comprises could be characterised as the substitution of patient confidence for the (benign) deceit and (sometimes) forlorn hope that currently characterise rationing by waiting in the NHS, with an acceptance by citizens that not all health care needs should automatically be satisfied by public resources. This approach would, therefore, have the further merit of providing a coherent role for the private sector. Queue jumping for important conditions would be reduced and the private sector could take over more of the work judged by the NHS – for whatever reason – to be 'low value'.

AN ALTERNATIVE

If this option is too radical – politically and technically – what can be done? In our view, the New Zealand initiative represents the right way forward. But it may be politically unrealistic to impose it nationally and for all conditions. As we have noted, despite a certain amount of technical work in various parts of the NHS, there has been very little effective debate on prioritisation as between patients or technical work on thresholds, and there remain strong disagreements about, for example, the role of cost in prioritisation. There is a pragmatic case for moving slowly.

This suggests two possible ways forward, which could in fact be combined:

- defining thresholds and times for a small number of important and common conditions such as cataract, joint replacement and CABG
- supporting local experiments in prioritisation through the development of scoring systems.

Currently PCGs are charged with adhering to national waiting list targets. Our proposal would be that these should be rejected in the present form entirely. They should be replaced by a mixture of national thresholds for specific conditions (as and when an evidence-based view as to where they should be set can be reached) and local choice over precisely what waiting time targets should be met and what level of activity should be funded, for other conditions.

Thus the national role should be redefined as supporting the exercise of choice at a local level, assessing or deriving the evidence relevant to determine priorities between patients and between treatments, and working with the wide range of measures that the Government has already initiated, to even-up standards in the execution of elective care itself. The national total waiting list would cease to be a target and, indeed, need not be published at all.

CONCLUSION

There is general agreement that the Government's emphasis on waiting lists measured at the time that patients are accepted for treatment is misplaced. There is less agreement as to what should be put in its place. Many have argued that the focus should be on waiting times. But while these are almost certainly too long for some conditions and should be shorter, waiting time targets do not in themselves provide the rationing mechanism required to ensure that the budget (whatever it is) is spent to best effect (however that is defined). Indeed, the tighter the waiting time targets, the more thresholds are needed to perform the rationing function.

At the political and rhetorical level, the main requirement is for a shift from waiting lists and overall waiting times to a broad commitment to equitable and appropriate access, combined with an explicit recognition that the NHS cannot 'do everything' – at least not immediately. The Government, stuck, at least for the time being, with its pre-Election promise to the people, seems unwilling to consider alternative policies. But if numbers waiting either for treatment or for consultation continue to rise, it may in the end be forced, as with Viagra, to confront the rationing issue.

REFERENCES

1. Frankel S, West S and R. *Rationing and Rationality in the National Health Service*. Macmillan, 1993.

2. National Audit Office. *Cataract Surgery in Scotland*. The Stationery Office, 1997.

3. Gray CS, Crabtree HL, O'Connell JE. Waiting in the dark: cataract surgery for old people. *BMJ* 1999; 318: 1367–68.

4. Harrison AJ, New B. *Access to Elective Care*. London: King's Fund (forthcoming).

5. Bridgewater B. Death on the waiting list for cardiac surgery. *Heart* 1999; 81: 564.

Viagra: the political management of rationing

Viagra has revitalised the NHS rationing debate, and has led to increased Government openness about the issue.

Steve Dewar

The decision by the Department of Health to restrict access to Viagra (Sildenafil) and other treatments for erectile dysfunction (ED) has raised important and fundamental questions about the essential task of rationing in the NHS. The decision by the Secretary of State highlights the complexity of the challenges posed by rationing. It also raises the technical and ethical problems inherent in making comparisons across different treatments and patient groups: who should gain, and who, by implication, should lose? And, importantly, how are such distributional judgements to be made? Who should be involved in such decisions, and how is a key stakeholder group – the public – to be engaged in rationing decisions?

Overarching all of these issues is the fraught political nature of rationing. When a new treatment is both clinically and cost-effective and the problem is appropriateness and affordability, the decision calls for social and political judgements. The Viagra decision is the first time the Secretary of State has led a major health care rationing decision. He has had to do this amidst a highly-charged atmosphere of conflicting political, public, professional and legal opinion, in a situation where not just money but information is a scarce commodity.

For health care professionals and managers rationing is a self-evident reality in the NHS. But for politicians in power it remains an extremely difficult issue to acknowledge. The Secretary of State explained his hesitancy to use the 'R' word in the House of Commons on 18 January 1999:

> *Those who want to make great political capital out of the rationing accusation are, by sleight-of-hand, trying to suggest that each patient is permitted only a fixed ration of health care or a fixed number of operations or drugs, regardless of his or her circumstances.*[1]

Whatever the truth of this assertion, it presented a particular definition of rationing that allowed Frank Dobson to state:

> *That sort of rationing is not happening and it never has. In the NHS, treatment is according to individual need, not pre-ordained entitlement.*[1]

Three days later the Secretary of State laid out proposals concerning treatments for ED that pre-ordained an entitlement for some and only exceptional entitlement for others. These proposals included access to treatment that was to be based not on individual need but on the presence of one of a number of underlying diagnoses for impotence.

So, difficult to acknowledge or not, the political decisions concerning Viagra suggest that politicians not only recognise the inevitability of rationing, but are also willing to grapple with the problem. Viagra thus represents an important political landmark in the history of the NHS. But how did it arise? And in particular, how was the decision managed?

CHRONOLOGY OF KEY EVENTS

First, what is the chronology of the key events in the Viagra story? Table 1 sets out the main events – from March 1998, when Viagra was granted market authorisation in the USA, to July 1999, when the Department of Health incorporated its final restrictions on access to treatments for ED into the regulations governing the NHS.* Early events were concerned with medical and scientific facts. Subsequently the political process took over the task of developing a policy that might survive public and professional consultation as well as legal challenge. Three elements of the process, looking to the facts, searching for guiding values and responding to the broader perspectives of others, form the structure of this article and are considered in turn.

TABLE 1

CHRONOLOGY OF KEY EVENTS IN THE VIAGRA STORY

	Key Events
March 98	*US market authorisation*
July 98	UK Government asks the Standing Medical Advisory Committee (SMAC) to prepare guidelines SMAC set up working party SMAC Chairman writes to Government, advising that Viagra should *not* be routinely prescribed until the Committee has finalised its advice
Sept. 98	*EU market authorisation* Government issues advice to doctors not to prescribe Viagra until further notice[2] BMA issues guidance advising doctors to follow the advice of SMAC as reported in the Government Circular
Nov. 98	Final advice from SMAC is made available to Government
Jan. 99	Prescription proposals for Viagra announced *with a six week consultation period*[3]
Feb. 99	Government Circular reminds health authorities that the advice to doctors not to prescribe Viagra is only *guidance*[4]
April 99	Consultation finishes – 861 replies received
May 1999	The Secretary of State announces the final decision[5] Pfizer wins its case – the original Government guidance in September 98 unlawfully sought to restrict prescribing
June 1999	A further Government Circular puts final restrictions into place within NHS legislation and advises GPs on frequency of prescribing [6,7]
July 1999	Restrictions on access to treatments for ED come into force

* GPs may issue NHS prescriptions to those men who in their clinical judgement are suffering from erectile dysfunction and have any of the following medical conditions: diabetes; multiple sclerosis; Parkinson's disease; poliomyelitis; prostate cancer; prostatectomy; radical pelvic surgery; renal failure treated by dialysis or transplant; severe pelvic injury; and spina bifida.

THE FACTS

The licensing process for any new drug treatment considers issues of safety, purity and effectiveness, but the NHS and its political masters also assess the evidence concerning cost-effectiveness and affordability. What are the facts in the Viagra case? And how were issues of cost-effectiveness and affordability weighed?

As the potential cost of Viagra became clear, ministers sought advice on key issues – cost, effectiveness and cost-effectiveness – from their medical and scientific advisers, in particular, the Standing Medical Advisory Committee (SMAC).* SMAC took advice from researchers at the University of Birmingham and evidence from Pfizer, the manufacturers of Viagra.[8]

TABLE 2

BASIC COST CALCULATIONS FOR VIAGRA

Example estimates from the recent literature

Population	*Prevalence (England)*	*Presentation*	*Appropriate*	*Frequency Prescribing*	*Price*
Total 49.3m Male 24m 20–75 = 16.8m 40–75 = 9.3m*	Complete ED for men aged 40–70: 5%–15% (average = 9.6%)[10]	Lower estimates of 38% of men with ED Upper estimate of 65% of men with ED[11]	70% of those presenting are appropriate for treatment, of whom 40% subsequently drop out[11]	50mg/once a week	Approx. £4.84/50mg dose

* Office for National Statistics

***A:** Numbers suffering ED*	***B:** The proportion who will present and appropriately require Viagra*	***C:** The annual unit cost of treatment*
• 2 million men (UK) with ED[12,13] • 1.75 million men (England) with ED[11] • Between 0.49 million* and 0.99 million† men (UK) with ED[14,15,10]	• 14%-17%‡[13] • 25%[14] • 27% §	• £312/yr per patient (including GP consultation cost)[11]

* Based on Kinsey (1948), used in National Prescribing Centre (1998).
† Based on Feldman (1994), used in National Prescribing Centre (1998).
‡ Of ED sufferers eligible for treatment within the proposals put out for consultation in January 1999.
§ Logical consequence of previous figures quoted in Burls (1998).

* SMAC has the task of advising government on medical issues. Since 1984 it has released more than 20 reports on topics such as the use of statins (1997), the use of donezepil (1998) and anti-microbial resistance (1998). Appointments to the committee are made by the Secretary of State for Health and members include the Chairman of the BMA and presidents of each Royal College.

The range of estimates for the cost of allowing unrestricted prescribing of Viagra within the NHS varied from £50 million to over £1000 million.[9] But why such a range of estimates?

Estimating the total cost to the NHS required information on a range of variables – population, prevalence, likelihood of presentation for treatment, likelihood of Viagra being prescribed, the frequency of treatment per patient and the eventual unit cost of Viagra to the NHS. Whilst some of this information is known, and known to be reasonably accurate, much is not. Table 2 presents various estimates for these variables using data from the recent medical literature, particularly figures from the University of Birmingham, the National Prescribing Centre, and the NHS Executive.

Estimates of the numbers of men suffering from ED show fourfold variation (500,000 to 2 million). The estimated proportion of sufferers who may present for treatment (and benefit from Viagra) varies from 14 per cent to 27 per cent. Unsurprisingly, such differences lead to wide variation in final cost estimates. Table 3 shows the range of costs assuming no restrictions on access to treatment, and presents some of the factors that confound efforts to reach an accurate answer.

Establishing even crude total costs is fraught with uncertainty, but the question of

TABLE 3

VARIABILITY IN BASIC COST CALCULATIONS AND POSSIBLE CONFOUNDING FACTORS

	Variability	*Confounding factors*
Numbers suffering ED	Fourfold variation.	Estimates vary according to definition of complete ED, source of prevalence estimates and use of population denominator.
Assumptions at the interface with services	Twofold variation.	Uncertainty concerning patient behaviour. A number of unanswered questions: • what proportion of those with ED want treatment? • what is known about the sexual behaviour and attitudes of older men? • what proportion of older men are sexually active? • how much will embarrassment prevent men seeking treatment? • what is the frequency of sexual intercourse for older men?
Total costs	• £38m to £77m* • £74m to £123m† • £50m‡	Crude estimates based on the price of prescribing ignore other important elements of cost. Full costs would need to consider the extent of changing patterns of workload in primary and secondary care, savings from changing treatments from existing interventions to Viagra and possible future physical and psychological benefits, particularly from earlier detection of underlying disease.

* Logical consequence of previous figures quoted in National Prescribing Centre (1998).
† Logical consequence of previous figures quoted in Burls (1998).
‡ Pfizer quoted in Brooks (1998) (*BMJ*).

affordability is even harder to pin down given that any calculation would need to take account of issues such as the changing patterns of workload for the treatment of ED in primary and secondary care, and the real savings to be generated from changing treatments from existing interventions to Viagra. Many of the elements of this equation are difficult to assess. Even the number of people receiving treatment for ED before Viagra became available is unknown. The University of Birmingham suggested that less than 10 per cent of men with ED seek medical treatment while the National Prescribing Centre stated that currently only 5 per cent of those with ED present for treatment.[14]

Per treatment, Viagra costs between 50 and 60 per cent of the cost of some of the existing treatments for ED – implying potential cost savings and/or higher treatment volumes within current expenditure. From the point of view of its clinical effects and management, Viagra is suitable for prescribing in primary care, has a lower side-effect profile, and does not routinely need specialist diagnosis and monitoring.[11]

So, Viagra turned out to be more effective, more acceptable and attractive to potential patients, and cheaper per treatment dose[11] than existing treatments for ED. However, despite the variation in estimates for the total potential cost, it also presented a probable problem of affordability – requiring either extra and new funding (or transfers from other areas of health expenditure) or some form of restriction on access (or perhaps a radical solution involving the exclusion of all ED treatment on the NHS).

The decision facing the NHS and its ministers over Viagra was complicated by the fact that men were already receiving treatment for ED. If the treatment of ED is to be part of the NHS, then the cheapness and effectiveness of Viagra meant that it had to be a main treatment option, otherwise the NHS would be ignoring principles of evidence-based practice and cost-effective prescribing. Disallowing a brand new treatment before it is used is one thing, taking away existing treatments is quite another.

Apart from excluding all ED treatments from the NHS, finding more money to accommodate Viagra or restricting access to keep within current expenditure on the ED budget, there was also a fourth option available – do nothing, and allow Viagra to reach its own level within the NHS, a level partly determined by clinical practice and partly constrained by the existing budgetary structure. This fourth option would essentially pass the rationing decision down to GPs and other clinicians. Examining recent experience of the muddle and confusion surrounding funding for the introduction of other, expensive, drug therapies (beta interferon), it may have been the case that the affordability issue was felt to be simply too large to devolve to a local level, or that a stand needed to be made against the 'postcode prescribing' that might have resulted. Whatever the argument, something had to be done, and extra funding was not going to be forthcoming.

But what was to be done and to what extent could clinical evidence be used to define restrictions on access? In their review of the data SMAC saw no *medical* reason why Viagra should not be available on the NHS for any man suffering ED. Nor did it find any obvious breakpoint, or step-changes, in the continuum of need for the drug.[16] If the facts had been slightly different the 'shape' of the decision may have changed. If there had been patients who were clearly in different classes of need, or if Viagra had different effectiveness profiles for clearly discernible patient groups, then such evidence may have formed the foundation for restricted access to treatment for ED. Such a restriction could have solved the affordability dilemma while providing a factual, medical and expert basis for targeted access in line with principles of effectiveness or greatest need. However, there was no way that restriction to treatment for ED could be based upon clearly distinguishable differences in need or effectiveness backed by medical fact.

It turns out that the type of decision demanded by Viagra was not amenable to a technical fix. As Richard Smith noted,

> *No expert can trade a man's impotence against a couple's infertility against adequate care for psychogeriatric patients against chemotherapy for childhood cancer. These trade-offs depend on the values of our society ...* [17]

Of course such trade-offs are made every day in the NHS. The real question is the ability of experts (or anyone else for that matter) to credibly justify such trade-offs in a way that is acceptable to all.

The Committee was clear that it was not its job to make recommendations concerning the affordability of health care innovations. Indeed, the Chairman went so far as to suggest that:

> *... the debate should include the ordinary man or woman in the street ... because it is the ordinary taxpayer whose money is being spent.* [18]

Ultimately, while recourse to the clinical and economic evidence helped illuminate the *type* of decision to be faced, such evidence had not pointed to a unique solution. In effect, SMAC handed the decision back to the politicians. As the Chair of SMAC explained at the time:

> *... the job of SMAC is to give medical guidance and medical facts to ministers on which they can make decisions. The ultimate decision is a political one in the widest sense.* [18]

So, on what basis did the Secretary of State make the decision to restrict treatments for ED within the current budget? How did he decide on an appropriate mechanism for restricting access to treatment? What were the values and criteria for these decisions? And on what basis could he have reached an answer?

GUIDING VALUES

From a technical point of view, the process of decision-making in the Viagra case appears to have followed the economist's practical approach to maximising efficiency: programme budgeting and marginal analysis (PBMA).[19] This technique essentially requires decision-makers to identify coherent programmes (of service) – such as treatment for impotence – to identify a budget for each programme, and assemble evidence of benefits arising from each programme. PBMA simplifies the complex task of comparing costs and benefits across services where the 'benefit' or outcome for each service is measured in units that are difficult to compare (lives saved, pain averted, etc.). The aim of PBMA is to maximise the efficient use of each programme budget; crudely, to reallocate within budgets until the greatest 'bang per buck' is achieved. This requires evidence not just of costs and benefits of current spending patterns, but alternative ways of spending the budget.

Setting the initial programme budget is a difficult task – but often current spending is taken as the initial starting point. This was the case with Viagra: the Secretary of State decided to define treatment for ED as the programme and accept current spending levels (around £10–£12 million) as the 'appropriate' spend for that programme. This was a decision about *allocative efficiency* – but no evidence was provided to support the decision, other than an appeal to the obvious superiority of 'programmes' such as cancer care, which dealt with life-threatening illnesses. Within the ED 'programme budget', the next decision to be taken was how much to invest in the new (and more effective) treatment – Viagra – compared with existing treatments. However, rather than defining an exact amount, the Secretary of State set access limits based largely on co-existing underlying disease that could cause ED. This effectively set an upper limit on the possible spend on Viagra. Having done this, the micro allocation decisions were passed to GPs and specialists to diagnose and treat in the usual way. It is clear that although such an approach is a rational (albeit rather utilitarian) way to bring transparency to such decision-making, the fact that this method was followed was not made explicit by the Secretary of State.[3]

So how does the decision on Viagra measure up? And against what values and criteria should it be tested? The Government has highlighted equity, fairness and transparency as appropriate values to guide 'prioritisation'.decisions. In July 1998, the then Health Minister, Alan Milburn, commented:

> *At the moment, decisions on how new treatments are introduced into the NHS whether they be drugs, interventions or new devices, are taken more or less on an ad hoc basis, usually at local rather than national level. ... This is why the Government has decided to set up the National Institute for Clinical Excellence ... The result will be greater national consistency.*[20]

The desire to move away from 'postcode prescribing' and towards greater geographical equity is clear. Proposals for appraising future health care innovations under the auspices of NICE reinforce this new emphasis that processes must be 'transparent and objective'.[21]

It is against these aspirations, alongside the different ways in which equity, fairness and openness are interpreted, that the decision should be examined. The final outcome meant that, for the first time, national guidance ensured that the same access rules applied across the country (notwithstanding some degree of difficulty in monitoring the actual application of these rules). However, while such national consistency is more equitable than the vagaries of 'postcode prescribing', it is perhaps arguable whether the imposition of a set of comparatively rigid access rules is the best application of basic notions of equity and fairness. For example, Calman has defined equity and equality in the following way:

> ***Equity*** *is about fairness and justice and implies that everyone should have an opportunity to attain their full potential for health.* ***Equality*** *is about comparisons between the level of health, or ability to obtain access to health care, of individuals and communities.*[22]

If equity means getting treatment appropriate to need then, in the case of Viagra, it is not possible to arrive at a solution that treats all needs equitably and does not break the budget. Given SMAC's view that, for Viagra, it is difficult if not impossible to identify clinical criteria for drawing a distinction between the needy and non-needy, then no national decision can be equitable in terms of satisfying the health care needs of all those men in equal need of care whilst at the same time respecting budgetary constraints.

Doyle has attempted to square this circle in proposals to guide rationing decisions whilst respecting the rights of each person to equal access on the basis of equal need and also acknowledging the scarcity of resources that make rationing inevitable.[23] He proposes that the budget for each specialty or health care programme be reduced by the same proportion in order to achieve the rationing required.

The basis for this argument is the need to maintain an equitable approach to the rationing of services in response to *all* health care needs. Doyle goes on to justify this position:

> *There is no acceptable moral justification for discrimination against particular types of treatment – against patients with specific clinical categories of disease and disability. Some illnesses will inevitably be more expensive to treat than others, and sometimes with less effect. Some will not find popularity with the public. Yet neither of these criteria can justify the denial or reduction of health care to those in need.*

Adopting Doyle's approach would represent a change in political and public attitudes given that some services are regarded as more important than others and are given different degrees of tragic status (at least by the press) depending on the illness or the sufferer. The equal moral status of different needs is not a commonly accepted notion in public debate. In the case of the decision concerning Viagra, the rationing burden has not been spread but met solely from within the notional budget (determined by pre-existing expenditure) for treating ED.

Alternatively, equity might be conceived of as the degree to which a rationing decision respects the different needs of *all those who want access to the full range of NHS services*. Certainly, the Secretary of State made it clear that some judgement about the worth of Viagra (and impotence in general?) versus all other services (and patient groups?) was made:

> *We have to find a sensible balance between treating men with a distressing condition, and protecting the resources of the NHS to deal with other patients, for example with cancer, heart disease and mental health problems.*[3]

The judgement that – at one extreme – life-threatening problems are more worthy of scarce NHS resources than non-life threatening illnesses is understandable; but there are many quality-of-life enhancing rather than life-saving treatments provided by the NHS – should the former always bow to the latter? The Secretary of State seems merely to have stated the initial rationing dilemma – that there are choices to be made – and elucidated one underlying principle for making a particular choice. But the nature of the 'sensible balance' is unclear; while comparison at the extreme is an attractive way of explaining a decision, only underlying criteria can inform future judgements between more similar classes of need.

But if – as many may agree – the treatment of impotence is not as important as treating cancer or heart disease, then what are the grounds for providing any treatment for impotence on the NHS at all? After all, the £12 million currently spent could easily be beneficially diverted to improving survival rates of cancer sufferers. Without consistent application of the Secretary of State's principle, political pragmatism and expediency may be seen as the guiding value. In this light the decision can be seen as taking a path of least resistance, working within existing expenditure and maintaining existing services as well as giving no hostages to future fortune.

While the outcome of a rationing decision may not be able to meet all the various and contradictory notions of equity, what about the *process* by which the decision was reached? That is, to what extent did the decision concerning Viagra adhere to some notion of *procedural justice*? A fair process might allow not only for openness, but also for clear rules that enable different propositions and interpretations of facts to be tested against known criteria. Such a process would enable those affected by the eventual decision to have some influence over the outcome; in other words, everyone can get his or her day in court.

Public consultation was in fact part of the Secretary of State's decision process. But there is, as Arnstein has noted, consultation that is empowering and consultation that may be tokenistic.[24] With many of the responses to the consultation questioning the rationale for using underlying diagnosis as a criterion for access to treatment for ED,[25] why did the eventual access restrictions retain such criteria? Why was the consultation set up so that it is not possible to review the 861 arguments presented?[5]

THE BROADER PERSPECTIVE

PBMA may have provided the technical framework for structuring the decision process with regard to Viagra, but there was (and is) a broader context into which this framework fitted (and was in turn influenced by). The *real politick* and context of the decision concerning the drug cannot be ignored – for example the extensive media coverage of Viagra, the nature of the problem the drug addressed and the nature of the drug itself, and the recent history of problems associated with the introduction of new and expensive drug therapies into the NHS.

In managing the Viagra decision through a highly-charged environment, a number of political tactics can be seen in action. The length of the process itself can be seen as one way in which the ground was prepared for the final decision. As early as September 1998 the Secretary of State signalled his determination that he would not allow demand for Viagra to lead to other patients 'being denied the treatment they need'[17] while still leaving the door open on any number of policy variations. This sort of statement allows the politician to test the water, and even at the time of the proposals for limited access to ED treatments (issued in January 1999) the consultation process enabled a postponement of any final calling to account for the decision. While the Secretary of State's proposals were criticised, the fact that the proposals were generally supported by media commentators[26] must have reassured the Secretary of State that the broad thrust of his decision would be acceptable to the public.

This cautious and staged approach does have the advantage that policy can develop within the public arena to fit the different pressures of public, professional and legal opinion. Lindbolm has described such an approach to policy development where positions are adopted and shifted over a period of time in order to try and accommodate the interests and values of other agencies or stakeholders.[27] His description of this process of policy development emphasises that a lack of transparency or clear values can have positive benefits. Without exposing underlying values, an assessment of the strength of a policy can be based on an 'agreement of the policy itself, which remains possible even when agreement on values is not'.[27] This pattern of incremental change and mutual adjustment fits in with situations where there are multiple pressures on policy development, and appears to describe the process of policy development in the Viagra case. However, this approach can seem somewhat arbitrary and fragmented. For example, Smith criticised the fact that policy on heath care rationing was being made 'piecemeal' and 'according to unknown criteria'.[17]

The main focus for criticism in the Viagra case was the lack of a clear set of evidence-based reasons for using particular rationing criteria (*viz.* the underlying diagnoses of men with impotence) as a way of restricting access. Whatever the lack of distinction between the needs of someone suffering ED with or without a particular diagnosis, the use of diagnoses as criteria for access to treatment implied a medical and scientific underpinning for the restrictions. In contrast to other options to restrict expenditure, the use of clinical criteria had the advantage (to ministers) of deflecting responsibility into worlds of technical, medical and scientific knowledge – worlds that are seen as closed to the majority of the public.

It also allowed the Government to use some aspects of the 'Viagra problem' to defend its position. For example, Viagra was seen in some quarters not as a serious drug therapy for a serious condition, but as a 'lifestyle drug' that could be used to increase sexual enjoyment for men not suffering from ED. This concern was fuelled by the lack of an objective test for ED and the media projection of an established recreational drug culture. The line against providing Viagra for those without ED was generally supported in the press and the position adopted by the Secretary of State that the NHS should not be 'financing people waving their potency at a disco' proved effective.[9] The impression that restrictions on access were required to stop such abuse helped justify the need to establish an underlying disease rather than accepting the 'legitimacy' of a psychogenic cause for ED.

While public opinion may be the final yardstick for the politician, the political decision had to have substance, and its successful implementation required clinicians to turn policy into practice. The fact that the manufacturers of Viagra, Pfizer Ltd, took a case against the Secretary of State's decision to court (arguing against his advice to doctors not to prescribe Viagra while substantive policy proposals were pending) is important for two reasons. First, because it shows how the pharmaceutical companies are now prepared to challenge government over the status of information that seeks to influence the behaviour of those professional groups working within the NHS. Secondly, because Pfizer's subsequent victory holds important lessons about the boundaries that determine the way government can manage clinical professionals in the NHS. These are lessons that will change the ways in which a system for more rational and explicit rationing develops.

The central point at stake in the court case was whether the Government had the power to impose a temporary ban on the prescription of Viagra, in apparent contravention of the requirement on NHS doctors to take clinical decisions in the best interests of their patients. It was accepted by all parties that the Government has the right to place restrictions upon prescribing through the use of a limited list of drugs (known by the legislation that established this right, 'Schedule 11' of the National Health Service Act 1977). But Mr Justice Collins (the judge in this case) indicated that the advice in the Circular of September 1998 should be struck down if 'the Circular was intended to and has achieved the same effect as if Viagra were placed in Schedule 11 and none of the safeguards or procedural requirements have been followed'.[28] In his opinion, this had been the case.

With regard to clinical freedom, Justice Collins concluded, 'it seems to me, the problem with the Circular is that the advice was given in a manner which meant that GPs would inevitably regard it as overriding their professional judgement'.

The implications are possibly far-reaching. It means that whatever the quality, reasoning or authority of any central guidance, ministers, the Department and the Executive of the NHS can only seek to inform and guide rather than override professional judgement on clinical matters unless – in the case of drug therapies – established statutory means such as Schedule 11 are used to limit clinical freedom. Following the outcome of the case, the NHSE issued a further Circluar,[6] which emphasised the guiding nature of the access restrictions and doctors' clinical duties towards their patients. But, to all intents and purposes, the access restrictions remained.

CONCLUSION

What are the lessons to be drawn from the Viagra story? The Viagra issue was not amenable to resolution solely through an analysis of data on clinical and cost-effectiveness. Rationing decisions such as this one raise questions of affordability that can only be resolved by weighing the relative priority that will be given to the treatment of different health care needs.

Proposals for the way that NICE might appraise new drugs stress that clear and authoritative comparisons of cost and clinical effectiveness are the key to the decision-making process. Suggested criteria for NICE appraisal include considering whether treatment should be 'targeted on groups who would derive most benefit'.[12] But this side-steps the difficulties that arise in cases such as Viagra, where the real issues are affordability and appropriateness. The NICE approach presupposes a clear differential in clinical effectiveness across a range of potential patients. In the case of Viagra this approach would not have been possible.

In these cases the Government proposes that NICE will make recommendations on the use of new health care innovation within the NHS and reach judgements on the value of new treatments relative to alternative uses of resources in the NHS. This seems set to happen *without* a clear role for politicians or the public in developing methods for addressing the very issues of affordability and comparative value of different health care programmes raised by treatments such as Viagra and considered by other 'expert' bodies such as SMAC as being beyond their remit.

Viagra raised problems at an awkward time. New Labour had already shown its hand against the perceived inequities of 'postcode prescribing', but the new National Institute for Clinical Excellence was still nothing more than a policy dream. So, the Secretary of State had to step into the breach. Many commentators have called for politicians to accept a role in making these decisions. However, it appears that there may be a potential mismatch between common tools of the politician's trade (where decisions invite agreement on ends rather than underlying principle) and the desire for a 'comprehensive, transparent and continuing debate that is based on evidence and values'.[17] The use of techniques such as consultation to manage a process of incremental policy development may not always promote greater equity, transparency or fairness.

The Secretary of State's decision seems to have been based on a programme budgeting and marginal analysis approach. But this emphasis on one particular approach to the rationing problem has its problems: not least the basic assumption that there is an existing budget for the treatment of a particular problem, or that this budget (often represented by current expenditure) represents some assessment of the priority placed on health in this area against any other area of need. In the case of Viagra the notional budget did not exist until it became the basis of the rationing decision. *Ad hoc* expenditure limited by the poor acceptability of previous treatments for ED became transformed into a budget representing the priority of treatment in one area against all others.

But what if the priority that experts, professionals or politicians want to put on a new area of technology actually means a change to existing expenditure and a consequential change in cross-programme budgets? It appears that the NHS is not organising itself to routinely consider this particular affordability problem. As different cases present different challenges to the existing pattern of access and expenditure there may be a need to move into this difficult territory.

The decision on Viagra shows that limiting access to ensure affordability can lead to problems. Asserting the value of life-saving treatments over interventions that enhance quality of life raises inconsistencies in existing patterns of expenditure. Where limited expenditure cannot be targeted according to criteria of need or effectiveness then the equity of outcome will be challenged. Meanwhile, the problem of finding a sound and open base for decisions that realign priorities and expenditure across programmes is still untouched by public debate.

The decision on Viagra did not substantially challenge the *status quo* – it maintained existing expenditure and access for those already receiving treatment. Even the use of medical criteria to justify restrictions to access rather misleadingly suggested clinical judgement at work. Indeed, the affordability problem was managed within the one health care programme involved. It may be that these parameters are not entirely a consequence of the particular questions posed by Viagra, but are partly influenced by the need to contain the potential difficulties that Viagra raised within policy solutions that were politically acceptable.

Future decisions might pose different problems, or the political imperative may change so that rationing decisions not only seek to ensure equity in terms of equal rules across the country, but seek to identify equitable rules that are equitably applied. In this case it might be advantageous to create the sort of environment where decisions that vary these parameters may also be acceptable. For this to happen the expert, the professional and the politician may need to believe that a range of conclusions are acceptable to the public and the Health Service. Only a wide debate will create the conditions necessary to make such flexible thinking possible.

New treatments or technologies that seek to move care into areas where previously there was no effective or acceptable approach will continually highlight this difficulty. Indeed, it would be logical for pharmaceutical companies to target areas of currently unmet high demand where need is difficult to assess or define. In this area new treatments will attract substantial direct marketing through the media and may flourish. The problems raised by this particular sub-set of rationing decisions will keep coming up. A new treatment for flu is on the horizon and raises a similar set of questions.

These problems will need to be tackled by NICE and will, like Viagra, require political direction over the allocation of public money. The experts and the politicians may need to make increasingly controversial decisions. However, it is difficult for politicians to lead this debate – they may prefer to follow rather than shape public opinion. NICE could be one organisation to help expand the range of acceptable decisions available to the politician by engaging the public in putting together a framework for rationing decisions and, thereby, helping to create the conditions for such open explanation and debate of health care rationing decisions – even by politicians. Such a framework could address the following questions:

- how can transparent comparisons of costs and effects across different health care programmes be made and explained?
- what role should politicians play in rationing decisions requiring decisions on how best to allocate public money for public good?
- what method of rationing or restricting access to clinically effective treatments on the grounds of overall affordability might be considered appropriate in different circumstances?
- how should the public be best involved in such decisions?

This increased openness will also be required as a consequence of the legal conclusions over the initial guidance on Viagra. Unless politicians use legislation to determine clinical practice they will need to make demonstrable arguments in order to influence behaviour. The judgement in this case has placed a high value on the need for those who wish to influence clinical decision-making to do so though open and sound argument rather than edict. This represents a challenge for political transparency and the ability of the decision-making process to handle both factual uncertainty and the unclear and varied values of many different stakeholders. For it is these facts and values that will help shape, determine and explain health care rationing decisions.

The story of Viagra shows that, while messy and difficult, it is possible to be more open when grappling with the difficulties of rationing.

REFERENCES

1. House of Commons Hansard Debates. 18 January 1999 (pt 12): Col. 589.

2. Department of Health. *Sildenafil (Viagra)*. Health Services Circular 1998/158. Leeds: Department of Health, 1998.

3. Department of Health press release 1999/0037. Consultation letter from Secretary of State for Health. *Treatment for Impotence*. Leeds: Department of Health, 1999.

4. Department of Health. *Sildenafil (Viagra)*. Health Services Circular 1999/042. Leeds: Department of Health, 1999.

5. Department of Health. *Treatment for Impotence*. Health Services Circular 1999/115. Leeds: Department of Health, 1999.

6. Department of Health. *Treatment for impotence*. Health Services Circular 1999/148. Leeds: Department of Health, 1999.

7. Department of Health press release 1999/0274. *Impotence Consultation –Dobson Announces Final Decision*. Leeds: Department of Health, 1999.

8. Department of Health press release 1998/377. *Interim Guidance on Viagra Issued*. Leeds: Department of Health, 1998.

9. Brooks A. Viagra is licensed in Europe but rationed in Britain. *BMJ* 1998; 317: 765.

10. Feldman HA, Goldstein I, Hatzichristou DG, Krane RJ, McKinlay JB. Impotence and its medical and psychosocial correlates: results of the Massachusetts Male Aging Study. *J Urol* 1994; 151(1): 54–61.

11. Burls A, Gold L, Simpson S, Clarke W, Stevens A. *Sildenafil: an oral drug for the treatment of male erectile dysfunction*. 1998 DPHE Report No. 12; InterDEC Report 28.

12. Booth A. Evidence-based practice digests: Topic: Sildenafil (Viagra) for erectile dysfunction. *Journal of Clinical Excellence* 1999; 1: 48–49.

13. Department of Health briefing notes BM No. 02/99. *NHS Prescription Proposals on Viagra*. Leeds: Department of Health, 1999.

14. National Prescribing Centre and UK Drug Information Pharmacists Group. *New Drugs in Clinical Development: Sildenafil*. Monograph Number 3/98/01. London: NHS Regional Office (South Thames), 1998.

15. Kinsey AC *et al. Sexual behaviour in the human male*. Philadelphia: WB Saunders, 1948: 236–237.

16. Johnson A. Letter of 9 November 1998 to Lady Hayman. The use of Sildenafil in the treatment of erectile dysfunction.

17. Smith R. Viagra and rationing. *BMJ* 1998; 317: 760–61.

18. Ferriman A, Harling R. The Man from SMAC. *BMJ* 1999; 318: 284.

19. Posnett J, Street A. Programme budgeting and marginal analysis: an approach to priority setting in need of refinement. *J Health Serv Res Policy* 1996; 1(3): 147–53.

20. House of Commons Hansard Debates. 14 July 1998 (pt 39): Cols 321–22.

21. Department of Health. *Faster Access to Modern Treatment: How NICE appraisal will work*. Leeds: NHS Executive, 1999.

22. Calman KC. Equity, poverty and health for all. *BMJ* 1997; 314: 1187.

23. Doyal L. Needs, right, and equity: moral quality in healthcare rationing. *Quality in Health Care* 1995; 4: 273–83.

24. Arnstein SR. A Ladder of Citizen Participation. *Journal of the American Planning Association* 1969; 35(4): 216–24.

25. Pownall M. UK consultation rejects restriction of impotence treatment funding. *BMJ* 1999; 318: 892.

26. Abbasi K. Viagra, rationed. *BMJ* 1999; 317: 765.

27. Lindblom CE. The Science of 'Muddling Through'. *Public Administration Review* 1959; 19: 79–88.

28. Judgement approved by the Court for handing down. *R. v. Secretary of State for Health, ex parte Pfizer Ltd.* Case No.: CO/4934/98. 26 May 1999, High Court of Justice, Queens Bench Division. Heard before the Honourable Mr Justice Collins, 10–11 May 1999.

The Modernisation Fund

The Government's commitment to improving the NHS has led to the creation of the Modernisation Fund. It is hoped that this injection of cash – along with political will and performance monitoring – will produce genuine benefits.

John Appleby

The 1998 Comprehensive Spending Review (CSR) – which has now replaced the old, annual Public Expenditure Survey (PES) – was the new Labour Government's first chance in nearly 20 years to get to grips with planning the totality of public spending and, importantly, to match spending with its manifesto commitments.[1] Not content with ditching the PES, the Government has also been busy reshaping the political lexicon. If there was one word that embodied the political rhetoric of new Labour, summed-up its political pledges (subliminally echoing the Party's new prefix) and simultaneously criticised the legacy of previous administrations, that word was 'modernisation'.

For health care the word is well chosen: the demand from patients tends to be for the latest, most up-to-date, cutting-edge treatment. In education, on the other hand, modernisation tends not to be what parents want for their children: 'new', in many people's educational terminology, goes with 'fangled'; and 'modern' goes with 'secondary' – commonly viewed as the very embodiment of failure and blighted lives.

So, modernisation in health care is good. But what, exactly, does it mean? And when the Government comes to put its (actually, our) modernisation money where its mouth is (though, unfortunately for dentistry, not literally) where does it go?

TOTAL SPENDING

Total spending on the NHS in England this year (1999/2000) is set to reach £39,703 million. Of this, £1163 million has been earmarked for the Health Modernisation Fund (HMF). This is equivalent to 2.9 per cent of the total budget (see Figure 1). Similar amounts have been allocated for the remaining two years of the current Parliament – bringing the total spend on modernisation to around £3 billion. As funding this year and next will be recurring – that is, built into the baseline budgets for subsequent years – the Treasury, somewhat unconventionally, describes the total spend as £5 billion. (If a similar accounting methodology had been used to describe changes in the NHS budget since 1948, spending today would be around £602 billion – about 75 per cent of GDP.) The HMF this year also represents over one-third of the cash increase in the total NHS budget between 1998/99, and over half the real (GDP-deflated) rise.

FIGURE 1

THE HEALTH MODERNISATION FUND: SHARE OF TOTAL NHS BUDGET 1999/2000

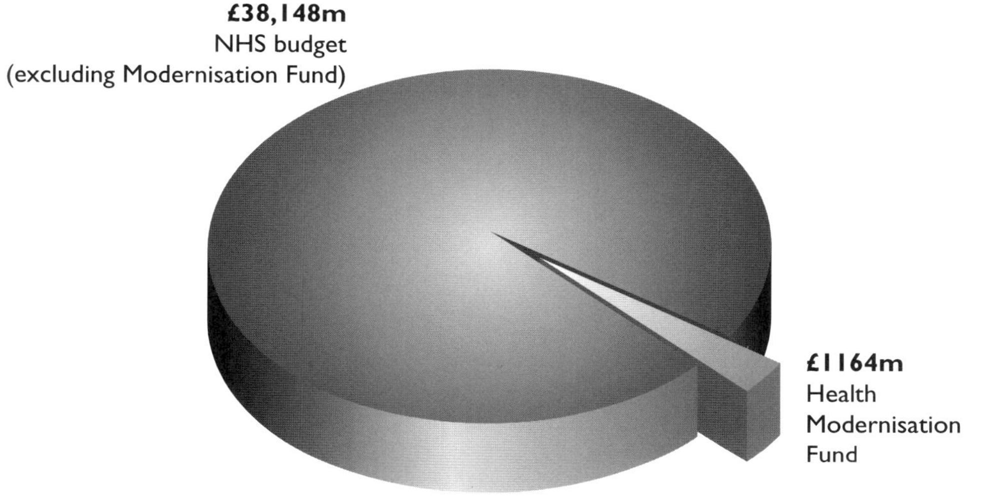

CSR AIMS FOR THE HMF

The Comprehensive Spending Review set out the Government's aims for the HMF (see Box 1):

Some of these aims are clear and achievements measurable – waiting lists for example. Others are somewhat vague: increased funding for health promotion – but how much? Increased training for NHS staff – but which staff, and what kind of increase?

BOX 1: AIMS OF THE MODERNISATION FUND

- **waiting lists:** to reduce numbers waiting to 100,000 below the level of March 1997
- **modernising hospitals and systems:** through the private finance initiative, and increasing publicly-funded capital by 50 per cent, to cut the number of mixed-sex wards and to buy new equipment
- **NHS staff:** to increase education, training and continuing professional development
- **mental health care:** to set up specialist community-based teams and increase spending generally
- **primary care:** to target additional funding for deprived areas, increase numbers of staff and improve practice premises and IT links to hospitals
- **health promotion:** to increase funding for health promotion and more community nurses

Source: Comprehensive Spending Review, p.47.[1]

ALLOCATING THE MODERNISATION FUND

In February 1999 the NHS Executive set out some of the details of how the Modernisation Fund is to be channelled into the NHS, and how it is to be spent.[2] Figure 2 shows the four allocation 'routes' to be taken by the HMF.

A comparatively small proportion of the HMF has been or will be allocated directly to *trusts* (primarily for the improvement of A&E departments and in the form of capital for tackling waiting lists). *Health authorities* will receive shares of the HMF, either through their main allocations or on the basis of specific plans – for example, to tackle long waiting lists. However, over half the HMF is held *centrally*, to be distributed in a variety of ways, such as to specific initiatives following bids either from health authorities/PCGs or in line with health authorities' main allocations.

None of these allocative mechanisms is particularly unusual: the Department of Health and the Executive have often retained part of the total NHS budget for redistribution to specific projects or to be spent on national schemes. More unusual, perhaps, is the scale of the funds either retained or handed over to the service and tied to planned developments approved by the centre.

INITIATIVES TO BE FUNDED BY THE MODERNISATION FUND

Bearing in mind that the HMF represents over half the real increase available to the NHS in 1999/2000, the degree of freedom for local commissioners and providers to make judgements about the use of the additional monies on the basis of local circumstances is somewhat limited. How limited becomes clearer on inspection of the individual service areas and initiatives to be funded from the HMF.

Figure 3 details the amounts to be distributed to various services and schemes from the HMF. Two areas absorb over half the HMF: waiting lists and waiting times (with waiting times increasingly appearing as a supplemental target), and primary care. Together with spending on staff development and medical and non-medical education and training, these areas account for three-quarters of the HMF.

FIGURE 2

FUNDING SOURCES FOR THE HEALTH MODERNISATION FUND 1999/2000

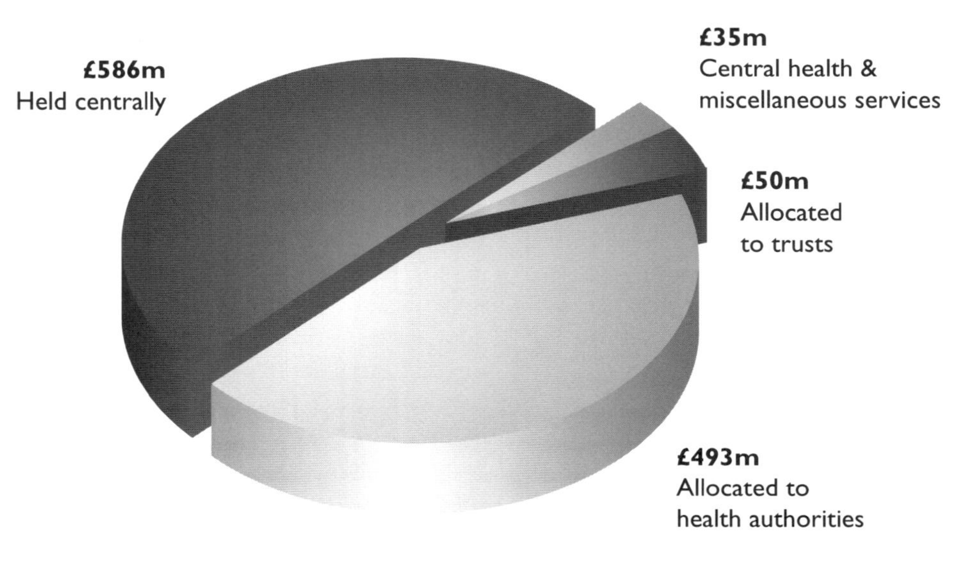

FIGURE 3

HEALTH MODERNISATION FUND SPENDING BY PROGRAMME 1999/2000

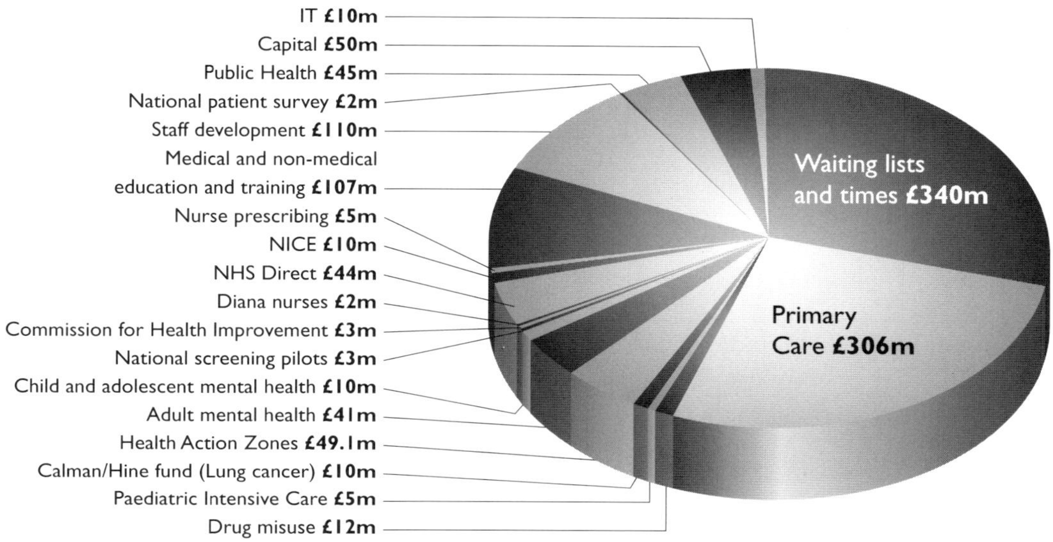

An important point to note is that the spending areas detailed in Figure 3 are not mutually exclusive: for example, while IT spending is shown as £10 million, there will be other spending on IT concealed within the spending in other areas (e.g. primary care). Accounting may be seen as a precise science but, as every accountant knows, a different story can be told simply by choosing a different basis upon which to present the accounts. On the face of it, primary care – a key priority area – is a significant beneficiary of money from the HMF. But, as Table 1 indicates, 44 per cent of the primary care element relates simply to the reallocation of the management allowance previously spent under the GP fundholding scheme; a further 13 per cent has been allocated for inflation for the general medical services budget and for the costs of closing down GP fundholding.

Similar accounting sleight-of-hand is detectable in the treatment of the monies allocated to staff development: £100 million (out of £110 million) is to be spent in support of 'recruitment and retention'. Very laudable, but this is just another way of saying that part of the costs of the 1999 Review Bodies' recommended pay awards will be funded from the HMF.

One could also query the inclusion in the HMF of spending to reduce the numbers on waiting lists: is this a particularly *modern* thing? Waiting lists (and times) have been an area of targeted, centrally allocated spending for many years.

So where does this leave the Modernisation Fund? Is it simply a bit of presentational rhetoric? Is it, rather, *post*-modern – an eclectic pastiche of previous, familiar spending initiatives? Or is it in fact just an old-fashioned device, beloved of exchequers everywhere, to try and ensure that it is possible to trace a connection between every extra pound they dole out and increases in the volume and efficiency of public services? The answer is probably yes to all of these: to believe that politicians are diffident people indifferent to the public perception of their policies, or that the Treasury takes a relaxed, *laissez-faire* attitude to the spending of

TABLE 1

MODERNISATION FUND SPENDING1999/2000

Programme area	*Comment*	*Health authority unified allocations*
Waiting lists and times	Reducing list sizes	260
	Performance fund and National Booked Admissions Programme	
	Cancer out-patient waits	
	Capital allocated to trusts to tackle waiting lists	
Primary care	Redeployment to PCGs of GPFH management allowance	135
	Cost of closing GPFH scheme	
	Other primary care initiatives (e.g. 'Beacons')	
	IT investment: allocated equally to all PCGs	
	IT investment: allocated on basis of relative need for IT	
	2.5% uplift to baseline GMSCL budgets for inflation	21
	Primary care infrastructure	58
	Second wave PCAPs	
	Out-of-hours doctor fund: inflation uplift	
	Out-of-hours doctors: additional funding	
	Implementation of GP Net	
Drug misuse	Distributed on the basis of drug misuse special allocation formula	
	Updating regional drug misuse databases	
Paediatric Intensive Care (PIC)	To fund a variety of PIC developments	
Calman/Hine fund (Lung cancer)	Implementation of Calman/Hine report recommendations	
Health Action Zones (HAZs)	Funding set up and running of HAZs	
	Funding developments in HAZs	
	HAZ innovation fund for deprived areas	
	HAZ evaluation and central support	
Adult mental health	Additional secure beds	
	Development fund	
	Beacon service Challenge Fund	
	24-hour staffed beds	9
	Assertive outreach teams	5
	Improving effectiveness of services	5
Child and adolescent mental health	Improving services: allocated on needs basis	
National screening pilots	Funding pilot sites	
Commission for Health Improvement	Set up and running costs	
Diana nurses	Funding Diana Children's Community Nurse Teams	
NHS Direct	Second wave pilot sites	
	Third wave sites and evaluation	
NICE	Set up and running costs	
Nurse prescribing	Implementation costs	
Medical and non-medical education and training	Funding for CPD, etc.	
Staff development	Recruitment and retention	
	Part funding of Review Body pay award for 1999/2000	
National patient survey	Funding of patient attitudes survey	
Public health	Development of public health capacity	
	Smoking cessation campaign: HAZ lead initiatives	
	Smoking cessation campaign: central initiatives	
	Mental health public health initiatives	
Capital	Improving A&E departments	
	Pathology	
	CHD National Service Framework	
IT	Funding for IM&T fund	
Total		493

Centrally funded initiatives, services and special allocations	*Central health and miscellaneous services*	*NHS trusts*	*Total*	*Programme total*
			260	
50			50	
10			10	
		20	20	**340**
			135	
19			19	
5			5	
10			10	
10			10	
			21	
3			61	
1			1	
2			2	
2			2	
40			40	**306**
11.9			11.9	
0.1			0.1	**12**
5			5	**5**
10			10	**10**
40			40	
2.6			2.6	
6			6	
0.5			0.5	**49.1**
14			14	
5			5	
2			2	
1			10	
			5	
			5	**41**
10			10	**10**
3			3	**3**
3			3	**3**
2			2	**2**
35			35	
9			9	**44**
10			10	**10**
5			5	**5**
107			107	**107**
10			10	
100			100	**110**
2			2	**2**
	24		24	
10			10	
	10		10	
	1		1	**45**
		30	30	
10			10	
10			10	**50**
10			10	**10**
586.1	35	50	**1164.1**	

other people's money is stretching credulity. The repackaging of a large slice of additional NHS funding is one thing; whether it produces the hoped-for service improvements is quite another. If it does – and experience suggests that targeted money combined with political will and performance monitoring does produce change – then the NHS should perhaps prepare for the next round of the CSR to deliver an expanded HMF mark II.

REFERENCES

1. HM Treasury. *Modern Public Services for Britain: Investing in reform: Comprehensive Spending Review: New Public Spending Plans 1999–2002.* Cm 4011. London: The Stationery Office, 1998.

2. NHS Executive. *Health and Personal Social Services Modernisation Fund.* Health Service Circular 1999/39. Leeds: NHSE, 1999.